THE
WAGES OF SIN

PETER LEWIS ALLEN

THE
WAGES OF SIN

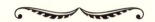

SEX AND DISEASE, PAST AND PRESENT

THE UNIVERSITY OF CHICAGO PRESS
CHICAGO AND LONDON

Peter Lewis Allen is the author of *The Art of Love: Amatory Fiction from Ovid to the "Romance of the Rose."*

The University of Chicago Press, Chicago 60637
The University of Chicago Press, Ltd., London
© 2000 by Peter Lewis Allen
All rights reserved. Published 2000
Printed in the United States of America
09 08 07 06 05 04 03 02 01 00   1 2 3 4 5
ISBN: 0-226-01460-6 (cloth)

Library of Congress Cataloging-in-Publication Data

Allen, Peter L., 1957–
    The wages of sin : sex and disease, past and present / Peter Lewis Allen.
       p.   cm.
    Includes bibliographical references and index.
    ISBN 0-226-01460-6 (cloth : alk. paper)
    1. Sexually transmitted diseases—Social aspects.   2. Sexually transmitted diseases—Moral and ethical aspects.   3. Sexually transmitted diseases—History.   4. Sexual ethics—History.   I. Title.
    RA644.V4 .A45 2000
    306.4′61—dc21   99-048603

♾ The paper used in this publication meets the minimum requirements of the American National Standard for Information Sciences—Permanence of Paper for Printed Library Materials, ANSI Z39.48–1992.

*T*o my mother,

Barbara Rapoport Taylor

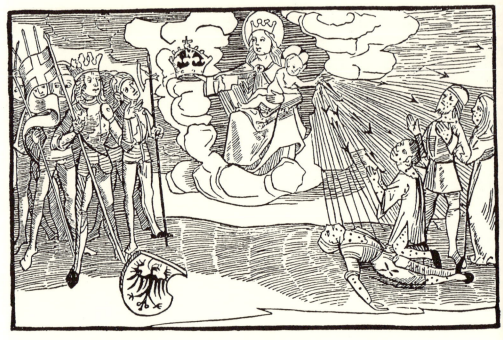

The arrows of syphilis. Woodcut from Joseph Grünpeck, *Treatise on the Pestilential Pox or French Disease* (Augsburg, 1496).

CONTENTS

ILLUSTRATIONS

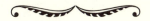

ACKNOWLEDGMENTS

There were times when I thought this book would never see the light of day. Above all, when things were rough, the person I would turn to was my friend and colleague Peggy Waller, who listened, read, advised, and encouraged throughout the years I have spent on this project. I am profoundly grateful to her.

Many other people also helped me along the way. Some went far beyond the call of duty: Sun Hee Kim Gertz, Bruce Schackman, and Monique Burke were exceptionally fine and conscientious readers. Victoria Harden took me under her wing; David Groff lent his extraordinary talents and experience in writing. My agent, Georges Borchardt, and my editor, Doug Mitchell, worked with me faithfully through many difficulties. My sister, Jennifer Taylor Fani, provided a skilled hand when it was most needed.

Others gave me assistance, food for thought, and support at every step. Some of the most generous were Mike Isbell, Derek Hodel, Ken Bowman, Michael Foreman, Katharine Park, Margo Amgott and Craig Stern, Peter Stanley, Quarry Pak, Debbie Cho, Gretchen Worden, David Calef, Mindy Finkelstein, Jeff Stryker, Dick Levinson, Bob Alig, Jonathan Mann, Cyrus Copeland, Paolo Fani, Vernon Rosario, Carolyn Dinshaw, Jerry Singerman, Joe McIlheny, Paul Bunten, Karen Reeds, Paul Farmer, Andrew Kirtzman, Danielle Jacquart, Michelle Minto, Carla Keirns, Daniel Tiffany, Bill Marsh, Jim Barlow, Robert Devens,

Carol Saller, Erin Hogan, the readers of the University of Chicago Press, and my students at Pomona College.

Generous grant support came from the Steele Foundation, the National Endowment for the Humanities, Pomona College, and the College of Physicians of Philadelphia. In addition, the staff and collections of many libraries were indispensable: the Bibliothèque Nationale, the Honnold Library of the Claremont Colleges, the New York Academy of Medicine, the College of Physicians of Philadelphia, the National Library of Medicine, the Wellcome Institute, Columbia University, the New York Public Library, Fordham University, and the University of Pennsylvania. The Gay Men's Health Crisis of New York kindly offered hospitality and resources, and the members of the departments of modern languages and literatures at Pomona College also gave generously of their insights and advice.

For interviews, I am indebted to Gary Bauer, Ron Bayer, Scott Burris, Art Caplan, Tom Coates, Jim Curran, Michael Foreman, Donald Francis, Helene Gayle, Mike Isbell, Harold Jaffe, C. Everett Koop, Art Leonard, Jeff Levi, Carol Levine, Martha Rogers, Theo Sandfort, Melissa Shepherd, Joseph Sonnabend, the late Tom Stoddard, and Jeff Stryker.

Finally, I would like to thank my mother, Barbara Taylor, for her love and support, and for always keeping me on the right track. This book is dedicated to her, and to the memory of all the people I have known and loved who have died of AIDS.

Introduction

THE FIFTH OF JUNE

If the American AIDS crisis had a birthday, it would be 5 June 1981. On that date, the Centers for Disease Control published an article about Pneumocystis pneumonia in its *Morbidity and Mortality Weekly Reports*. In this short piece, two UCLA doctors announced that they had found a number of cases of this highly unusual disease among some of their gay male patients in Los Angeles. For epidemiologists, this little article would come to be the shot heard 'round the world—the first public warning of a disease that would take millions and millions of lives.

I knew nothing, however, about all this. June 5 was my twenty-fourth birthday, a pleasant spring day I spent doing research in the medieval and Renaissance collections of the Newberry Library in Chicago—an appropriate way, I thought, to begin a year in which I aimed to make significant advances in my scholarly career. Overall, this was a happy time for me. I was completing my Ph.D. coursework at the University of Chicago; I would be spending the coming year at the medieval studies center in Poitiers, France, on a graduate fellowship; and I was living with my lover, a handsome young Scotsman named Stewart Telfer whom I had met while spending my junior year in Aberdeen four years before.

Despite all these good things, however, not everything in my life was peaceful. Stewart and I loved each other very much, but each of us was pulled away by outside interests—his in other men, mine in my work, which was so important to me I was about to set off for ten months in France, hoping that when I returned I would somehow find our problems magically resolved. I was wrong, but not in a way I could have predicted on that balmy day I spent in the library, looking forward to a celebratory dinner later on.

I left for France that August and returned the following May, a little bruised by unforgiving Gallic professors but holding a French graduate degree and ready to pick up domestic life as I plunged into the final stretch of my doctorate. Almost as soon as I had set foot on American soil, however, Stewart informed me that he no longer wanted us to be a couple.

The pain of our separation turned my emotional life upside down, but even as I adjusted to it, a bigger shock followed. The gay papers and some of my better connected friends were spreading rumors about a new disease racing through the fast-lane coastal cities of New York, San Francisco, and L.A. Nobody knew much about it, other than that it seemed to have something to do with gay men and sex; the little we did hear was confusing and contradictory. Some authorities warned us to avoid poppers (inhaled amyl nitrate); others said that all we needed to do to stay safe was to know our partners. One friend's doctor told him to avoid sex until the whole thing blew over—advice that seemed ridiculous to the rest of us. Now I wonder whether my friend took that advice—and whether he's still alive. To me, it seemed that San Francisco was a long way off, and that its troubles were unlikely to affect us in the safe haven of the American Midwest.

Fifteen years later, almost all my closest associates from my Chicago days are gone: Stewart; our close friend Michael Botkin and his lover, Joe Alongi; Michael's best friend, Andy Leo; friends and lovers of friends—the list goes on and on. There was no safe haven from AIDS—not in the Midwest, not in any region of the United States, nor in any country in the world. By the middle of 1999, 711,344 Americans had been diagnosed with AIDS, and 420,201 of them had died. And despite major advances in treatment, the rate of new infections has not slowed; in fact, it rose 10 percent in 1998. Half of all new infections, both in the United States and around the world, are in people under twenty-five. Worldwide, 16,000 people are infected with HIV per day—a total of 5.8 million in 1998. In certain parts of Africa, one in four adults is HIV-positive.[1] Studies in 1999 predicted that 40 million people would be living with AIDS by the year 2000. Since the pandemic began, more than 48 million adults have been infected; more than 14 million of them are dead.[2]

No one can bear witness to more than a small part of the story of AIDS. My part began with Stewart, then expanded beyond him into the historical exploration that became this book. The lessons I learned in my own life, through my relationship with one individual, turned out to hold a greater truth: that, in its fights about how to respond to AIDS, American society was reenacting a drama that had been written centuries before. I learned that there was a long tradition in the West of seeing disease as God's punishment for sin—especially for sexual sins. I learned that every era had sorry tales to tell about how the sick and dying were condemned for their illnesses, and made to suffer as much in mind and heart as they were suffering in their bodies. I learned of the deep-seated conflicts in the great traditions of medicine and religion—the conflicts between compassion and condemnation, healing and blame. And I learned that despite America's apparent modernity, many people in this country—including many of those in power—were convinced that the healthy were saved and the sick were damned. All of these things, I found—history, conflict, condemnation—directly affected the course of this new epidemic, and took an enormous and tragic toll on Americans' health and lives.

Stewart taught me these lessons in several ways. I learned them through the sad and frightening day-to-day experiences of having a close friend undergo the rigors of this torturous disease—repeated hospitalizations, endless drug regimens, pneumonia, shingles, CMV blindness, wasting, dementia. Through Stewart's background and experience, I also learned about parts of Western culture that had been very foreign to my experience. I learned that repressive attitudes about sex and sin that I thought had been left behind for decades, if not centuries, were actually vigorous and widespread in my country and were having drastic effects on my life and the lives of many people I knew.

The rhetoric of the Christian right, which would become so familiar to America with the advent of the Reagan era, was hardly news to Stewart. He had grown up on a sheep farm so rural that it did not get electricity until 1964, in a family whose lineage was replete with ministers and missionaries. As a teenager, Stewart himself had embraced conservative Christianity, selling Bibles door-to-door in France, serving as the prayer secretary to the University Christian Union, and choosing a career in the Presbyterian ministry. When I met him at the University of Aberdeen, Stewart was a third-year student in divinity. Part of his religious leaning was an outgrowth of his background, but another part was a way of running away from being gay, an orientation he alternately lived and fought against. The homosexual life Stewart had found in the Scottish provinces in the 1960s and 1970s was, not surprisingly, composed of equal parts shadow, intrigue, risk, and shame. The stories he told me were peopled by such characters as Sandy, the "town queer"; the occasional American tourist; the odd assortment of flora and fauna that inhabited Aberdeen's two gay bars; a policeman in a men's restroom who warned him against public sex; and a very discreet circle of gay ministers in the Church of Scotland. Same-sex relationships were not absent from this old-fashioned world, but they were infused by the belief that sex was bad, homosexuality was worse, and that whatever was sinful would be duly and visibly punished.

Like an asteroid, I fell into Stewart's life in January 1977 during my junior year abroad—a Reform Jew from the Upper West Side of Manhattan, a member of a family that voted a straight Democratic ticket and viewed Saturday services with far less religious awe than we did the Sunday *New York Times.* During my sophomore year at a Quaker liberal arts college, I had come out as a gay man, and I now was determined to preach my new social gospel to the twenty-one-year-old redhead who, by March, was spending more and more evenings at my table and in my bed. We spent almost as much time arguing about religion and morality as we did making love.

That August I returned to the States to complete my senior year, while Stewart went back from his parents' farm to Aberdeen to finish his. The day after he graduated, he said good-bye to his family and got on a plane in Glasgow; six hours later I picked him up at JFK. In New York and Chicago, we lived together for three years amidst the joys and pains of more-or-less married gay life, a life rendered even more complicated by the differences in our backgrounds and by our youth. When we separated in the summer of 1982, I spent the summer in a flood of tears and moved reluctantly to a place of my own.

That move broke my heart, but it probably saved my life: just around this time, we later figured, Stewart was infected with HIV. As time went on, we grew apart in some ways. I moved to New Jersey, and then to L.A.; each of us moved on to relationships with other men. But we also remained bound together at heart by years of love and our struggle to deal with his disease. As the 1980s hastened on, Stewart grew thin and frail; gradually, pieces of his mind began to slip away, though he never lost his wisdom or his dignity. I visited several times a year, and kept in frequent touch by phone, each contact a step further down the path to his journey's end. "I have to go now," he told me at the end of one short and dreamlike telephone conversation in early 1990, and I knew that what he was telling me was true. Despite all the love and care his friends and health care providers could offer, he withered, and on May 23 Stewart died, held close by his new lover, Ira Johnson, and me.

SILENCE = DEATH

When I was not preoccupied by sadness in these years, I watched the AIDS crisis being played out on the larger, national stage, and I could not help feeling that things were going just as badly there as they were in my own life. Above all, an uncanny silence about AIDS spread over the country, a kind of sonic and emotional black hole into which the anger and grief of those who were suffering fell without resonance or response. Presidents Reagan and Bush, much of Congress, and most of the mainstream media simply looked the other way. Most of my family, my teaching colleagues, and my heterosexual friends were quiet, too, either because they did not notice what was happening or—more probably—because they did not know how to ask. Immersed in continuing losses, I scarcely knew how to talk about them. When people asked me how I was, I rarely had the strength of heart to admit my grief, despair, and fear; overwhelmed, I just let the stillness grow thicker, undisturbed.

When there *was* public noise about AIDS, it was even more disturbing than the silence. From some of the more vehement conservatives in Congress, from the White House staff, and from the prominent preachers on the religious right who were distilling venom into the nation's ear came threats of fire and damnation that shocked even Calvinist Stewart and dumbfounded and infuriated me. I was completely bewildered that people who called themselves Christians—whose religion claimed to be based on healing and compassion—could be blaming this terrible disease on the gay men who were suffering and dying from it.

Even more amazing to me was the fact that the sentiments of these zealots were echoed by some members of the medical community. Early on in the epidemic, when Stewart was working at a job he had found at the American Society of Clinical Pathologists, he called me one evening, in tears. "One of the doctors at work today," he told me, "called AIDS the 'Wrath of God Disease.'" Haunted as Stewart was by the ghosts of his fundamentalist past and his fears about his own health, this remark had left him frightened and angry.

This callous pathologist was scarcely alone in his views. A 1984 editorial in the official journal of the Southern Medical Association, entitled "Homosexuality: Kick and Kickback," reasoned that AIDS was

God's punishment for gay men's sins—"the due penalty of their error," the editor explained, quoting St. Paul.[3] Elsewhere, an anonymous surgeon put matters this way: "We used to hate faggots on an emotional basis. Now we have a good reason."[4] Substantial numbers of physicians agreed: a 1991 survey of U.S. doctors revealed that half of them would refuse to treat people with AIDS if they could, and nearly a third thought there was nothing wrong with this response. Promiscuous homosexuals and drug addicts, in these doctors' eyes, were simply bad patients—patients they had no responsibility to help.[5]

MEDIEVAL ROOTS

Time and again, I found myself wondering, "Why are these people talking this way about AIDS?" And because I tend to look to origins for explanations—a preoccupation that had led me to a professional training in classical and medieval literature—I began to guess that these attitudes had roots deep in Western culture. Bit by bit, my academic research began to confirm these suspicions.

Not long after Stewart died, I read a book by a Stanford scholar, Mary Frances Wack, entitled *Lovesickness in the Middle Ages*. It recorded the history of a strange disease that had apparently been a standard topic in the medical textbooks of the Greek, Arabic, and European world for more than a thousand years. The symptoms of "lovesickness" ranged from mild (irregular pulse, loss of appetite, mental preoccupation) to weird (some medieval writers said that the disease could turn men into werewolves) to dire (insanity and death). Even more peculiar than the idea that love could be considered an illness were the cures these physicians prescribed. Some doctors recommended herbal and psychological remedies, and others the painful but standard premodern practice of drawing off excessive blood from the patient's veins. Not a few, however, recommended a cure that quickly seized hold of *my* imagination: sexual intercourse, they asserted, would relieve the system's imbalances and restore the patient's body and mind to health. Startlingly, these doctors did not seem to care much whether their patients were married to their sexual partners or not—especially if the patients were men. In what had, since antiquity, been seen as a simple matter of health, marriage was not a primary concern. The prescription for sex, in other words, could be filled at any pharmacy that would honor it.

Wack had not drawn any explicit connections between this odd medieval phenomenon and the deadly epidemic that was racing through

America, but, surrounded by AIDS as I was, I could scarcely *not* see links between the social implications of these two diseases. The European Middle Ages, I knew, had given birth to such central cultural institutions as the Church, the university, and the medical school, and even the nation-state. As the late scholar Paul Zumthor observed, the Middle Ages was the cradle of the modern world.

On a study leave from my West Coast teaching position in Paris in 1992, I began to follow my curiosity through the amazing collections of the Bibliothèque Nationale, and bit by bit I found evidence that the past and the present did have significant parallels in the areas I was studying. Mary Wack's history of lovesickness was quite accurate, but it did not answer questions I had about the way in which this peculiar disease and its even stranger remedy had been viewed by the Catholic Church, an institution that had made its influence felt in nearly every aspect of medieval European life. If twentieth-century cardinals and ministers felt that using condoms in AIDS prevention was a sin, I thought, it would be truly amazing if their medieval forbears had let lovesick patients commit fornication or adultery just because their doctors told them to. Sure enough, what I had suspected was true: medieval churchmen had not seen eye-to-eye with their medical counterparts in this regard. For the ecclesiastics, in whose scales the soul weighed far more heavily than its fleshly shell, the sin of wayward intercourse was so grave that it was better to let the patient die from lovesickness than to fornicate and be cured but in the process consign his or her soul to the everlasting torments of hell. The classical and Islamic traditions out of which medieval academic medicine arose, however, paid little attention to these spiritual concerns: for them, it was the physician's job to do what was necessary to heal the body, while the rest lay outside their domain. The gap between the medical and religious views of lovesickness contained the ideas that would become the present book.

Rather than look only at the Middle Ages and compare it with the present, I decided to see whether I could find a trail between them—a tradition of beliefs, attitudes, and examples that had something in common with lovesickness and AIDS. Following the advice of friends and colleagues, I searched through many libraries and hundreds of books, and ultimately assembled a cluster of diseases that, in their day, had been closely linked with sin. The results of that search form the chapters that follow—on lovesickness and leprosy in the Middle Ages, syphilis in the Renaissance, bubonic plague in seventeenth-century England, medical treatments for masturbation in the eighteenth and nineteenth centuries, and, finally AIDS. A frightening but fascinating story emerges from the pages that follow: the story of the idea that these diseases were punishments for sinful behavior. The only sure way to avoid sickness, this thinking went, was to avoid sin. As the English author Thomas Dekker advised his countrymen in 1630, in the face of bubonic plague, "Only this antidote apply: Cease vexing Heaven, and cease to die." The consequences of this belief have been grave: the sick have often been subjected to society's scorn and fear, and prevention has often been neglected, on the principle that it was immoral to teach people how to avoid a disease transmitted by something they should not have been doing in the first place.

Some of the stories I turned up are extraordinarily sad, like those of medieval lepers pronounced dead to the world and forced to wander and beg a meager living, stigmatized by red badges, incurable and disabled, and forbidden to touch or even speak to another human being. Many are shocking, either because of the painful and repugnant symptoms (the blackened and deadly swellings of bubonic plague and the rubbery, suppurating tumors of syphilis) that the sick experienced or because of the unkindness with which they were treated. For me, these images were often matched in cruelty by the attitudes of the healthy, many of whom saw themselves as enforcers of morality: the medieval administrators who expelled pregnant lepers from their hospices, for example, or the French aristocrat Marie de Maupeou Fouquet, whose 1678 book of home remedies observed that the ugly origin of venereal diseases made them the "just effects and temporal chastisements" of lust, that deadliest of sins. This author distinguished "innocent" from "guilty" victims three hundred years before a similar pronouncement from self-proclaimed AIDS martyr Kimberly Bergalis. Far from giving aid to the guilty victims of syphilis, Mme. Fouquet coldly observed, "we should increase their sufferings and mete out to them rigorous penances rather than easy remedies."[6]

As this seventeenth-century language shows, accusations and condemnations were not limited to ecclesiastics: as in the case of AIDS, the sick were often criticized by lay and professional medical authorities, too. Some authors chose not to publish remedies for these reprehensible diseases; others administered treatments (often completely ineffective) that were as bad as what they purported to cure. Renaissance physicians, for example, were fond of sending their syphilitic patients to sit in mercury-vapor steam baths until the toxic fumes caused the unfortunates to emit a quart of saliva a day, often losing their teeth in the process; sometimes the patients died.[7] Nineteenth-century physicians and surgeons were even crueler in trying to keep their patients from the dreaded habit of "onanism": these doctors confined men, women, and children in straitjackets, cauterized them with red-hot irons, circumcised them without anesthetics, or even cut off clitorises and testicles altogether. Terrified by a "disease" they thought would make them crazy or kill them outright, many patients cooperated in these gruesome procedures as a preventive measure, or even sought them out. (One day, perhaps, such modern treatments as chemotherapy and radiation may join this list. As medicine changes, old practices quickly come to seem equally barbarous.)

These grim stories have been counterbalanced by inspiring examples of kindness in both the medical and religious traditions. Greek, Roman, Jewish, Moslem, and Christian physicians dedicated their lives to healing. Cure and compassion have been central to religion, as well—especially Christianity, whose early success was based in good part on miraculous cures, even of the diseased and outcast. Jesus himself healed many people—the blind man by the Jericho road in the Gospel of Mark, the lepers in the book of Luke, the epileptic demoniac of Matthew 17, and even the greatest healing act of all, recorded by John: raising Lazarus from the dead. Following in Christ's path, St. Basil of Caesarea (ca. 330–379A.D.) founded the West's first hospital, in which he personally attended to the sick poor. The tradition he began gave rise to vast networks of care in Byzantium, in the Islamic Middle East, and in Europe. Catholic and, later, Protestant physicians drew inspiration from this rich heritage, and their successors make it live today, both in the many modern hospitals of religious foundation and in the principled and courageous works of individual Christian doctors such as former surgeon general C. Everett Koop. In my research, interviews, and writing, I have come to a far greater understanding of and respect for Christianity than I had before. Yet I remain even more troubled when Christians have failed to live up to what I see as their religion's greatest strengths—its ideals of equality, humility, empathy, and charity.

THE FINE PRINT

At times I have found myself trying to write a book that told the entire story of sin and disease in Western culture over the past two thousand years; fortunately, these lapses from reason have been brief. Instead of this impossible task, I have tried to present these pieces of the past in a way that would make sense and illustrate the commonalities between then and now without making generalizations I could not support or that were simply untrue.

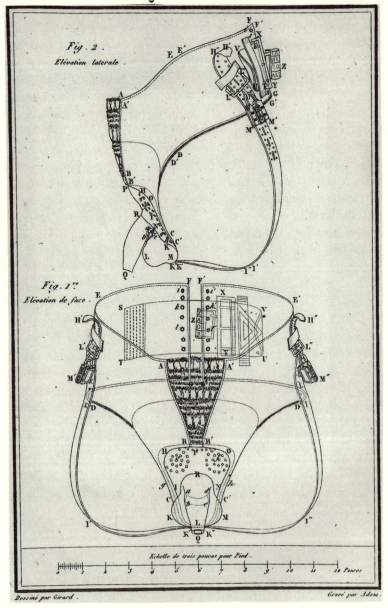

Antimasturbation truss. From G. Jalade-Lafond, M. D., *Considerations on the Preparation of Corsets and Belts Designed to Oppose the Pernicious Habit of Onanism* (Paris, 1819). Courtesy of the Wellcome Institute Library, London.

The result is not a continuous history, but rather a series of portraits of disease arranged in rough chronological order. Individually, these stories open windows onto a particular era and the conditions that surrounded a disease at that time. Together, I hope they create a perspective on the European and American scene from the Middle Ages to the present—a tableau that I believe is more than the sum of its parts. What *I* see from this perspective is a continually changing yet persistent culture in which various institutions have struggled with conflicting values in their attempts to understand, explain, and come to terms with the fundamental human experiences of sexuality and disease. I have not tried to eliminate my personal views from my writing because I felt that there was no way to make a book such as this totally objective. Instead, the book is a mixture of personal experience and scholarly research that I hope will help its readers become aware of the huge cost of seeing disease as a punishment for sin.

I have two disclaimers to make. One is that I am not an expert in many of the fields this book covers, and even seven years of diligent study are far from enough to have made me into one; despite my efforts, the book will contain some errors of fact and interpretation, and I apologize for these. The other, equally important, is that I am not a historian but a literary scholar—a professional reader trained in finding and making meaning in texts. A crucial part of my education was the process of learning that meaning is *always* subjective—that what we see depends on who we are and how we look at the world. I hope that you, my reader, will start by letting me be your guide in what is likely to be unfamiliar terrain. Gradually, as you learn more about the subject, and as my narrative reaches more modern and familiar ground, I invite you to turn this method of finding meaning both on the book you hold in your hands and on the larger and more significant text of the present-day world and the ways in which we try to understand its myriad events.

Perhaps the best way to explain my hopes for the book you are about to read is to borrow the words of Thomas Vincent (1634–1678), the author of *God's Terrible Voice in the City,* an extraordinary narrative about the outbreak of plague in London in 1665. "If it were fit," Vincent wrote,

> I would begin here with myself . . . and I would beseech every one of you that cast your eyes upon these lines, to do the like, and to compare them with those lines which are written in the Book of your consciences; and where you do find a transcript, read and read again, consider and lay to heart.[8]

CHAPTER ONE

Sex by Prescription: Lovesickness in the Middle Ages

In his annals of the history of England, Roger de Hoveden (d. 1201?) recorded the following curious entry. On Tuesday, February 24, of the year 1114, wrote Roger,

> Thomas the Younger, Archbishop of York, departed this life. When he was first taken ill, his medical men told him that he could not recover, except by means of carnal knowledge of a woman. On which he made answer, "Shame upon a malady which requires sensuality for its cure!" And being thus chosen by the Lord while of virgin purity closed his temporal life.[1]

The historical record contains a few other details about Thomas—that he came from an ecclesiastical family; that he was good-natured and an eloquent speaker; that he had been entangled in a complex investiture debate; and that he was enormously fat.[2] But what about the malady that required sensuality for its cure?

Any twelfth-century physician—indeed, almost any physician from the second century to the eighteenth—would quickly have recognized that Archbishop Thomas was suffering from lovesickness. This disease was decidedly one of the stranger novelties in the Renaissance of the twelfth century, a period when knowledge from classical Greece and Rome and the Islamic world was pouring into Christian Europe at an unprecedented rate. Much of this information explosion—the observations and speculations of the pagan philosophers and heathen scientists, not to mention the classical poets' immoral fictions about the sexual escapades of the pagan gods—was troubling enough to the more conservative parts of the Church. But lovesickness raised problems that were graver still.

Physicians believed that lovesickness was a kind of melancholia (in modern terms, depression), caused by an excess of black bile, a thick, sluggish humor responsible for many disorders of the brain. If a person fell in love with someone who did not return his or her affections, or simply abstained from sex for too many weeks or months, black bile would build up in the body and cause all kinds of mental and physical ills. First came severe emotional instability. A beautiful face, for example, would send the affected person into fits of excitement or a murderous rage, according to the Persian physician-philosopher Avicenna (Abū ʿAli Husayn ibn-ʾAbdullāh ibn Sīna, 980–1037); the patient would fluctuate between sparkling hilarity and deep grief. Love songs would make the unfortunate sufferer weep; at other times, the patient's eyes would be sunken and abnormally dry, the eyelids fluttering as if in response to a scene that no one else could see. The mere thought of the beloved would cause violent irregularities of the pulse—a sign that alerted insightful doctors to what might be wrong.

If the disease remained untreated, more severe symptoms were sure to follow: the lovesick could not sleep, they became distracted, they grew pale. Their sexual desires raged out of control. Constantine the African (ca. 1020–1087; a noted Arabic scholar turned Christian monk) and Peter of Spain (1220?–1277, the future Pope John XXI), noted that sometimes the patient's skin turned yellow, taking on a jaundiced cast. The Persian Rhazes (Abū Bakr Muhammad ibn Zakariyyā al-Rāzī, 865–925), considered the greatest clinician of the Moslem world, had noted that the most severely afflicted sometimes displayed the mark of doglike bites on their faces, backs, and legs, and might even turn into werewolves, marauding through cemeteries by night. As the disease progressed, wrote Bernard of Gordon (fl. 1285–1308, a professor at the prestigious medical school of the University of Montpellier), "the prognosis is such that unless the lovesick are helped, they fall into madness or die."

The Church might have ignored these complaints: after all, what was one more disease in this sad world? But lovesickness had one feature that made it both unusual and deeply morally problematic: doctors claimed that lovesickness could be cured by sex. Their logic was inexorable: if the disease was caused by a buildup of black bile and its byproducts, "atrabilious" blood and semen, the simplest and most effective way to relieve the suffering patient was to void these fluids from the body. Bloodletting was one good cure; equally effective was another process of evacuation: sexual intercourse. The patient's partner hardly mattered; in fact, it scarcely made a difference whether there was a partner at all. The important thing was to get the toxins out.

MANAGING THE BODY, AND THE "ACCIDENTS OF THE SOUL"

The logic of lovesickness and its treatment derived from the concept of the four humors, a doctrine that dated back to classical Greek theorizing that everything in the universe was made up of four elements—air, fire, water, and earth. Within the human body, character and health were determined by a parallel pattern of four fluids, or humors (blood, red bile, black bile, and phlegm) as they ebbed and flowed. Hippocrates (ca. 460–377 B.C.), the most influential early medical figure in classical Greece, rejected earlier notions that diseases were punishments sent by the gods; instead, he attributed illness to an imbalance of these fluids, a disequilibrium that caused disease and pain. A good physician, the Hippocratic writings explained, restored his patient to health by balancing the humors in accordance with the individual's temperament, the seasons, and the disposition of the stars. To modify these internal, "natural" operations, the doctor would regulate the external, "non-natural" behaviors he could control: "air, exercise and rest, sleep and waking, food and drink, and the 'accidents of the soul,' or passions and emotions."[3] Managing the patient's sleep, exercise, and diet, and drawing off excessive blood, menses, and even the male and female seed[4]—these were the procedures classical medicine used to restore invalids to health.

The structure of classical society made it possible to include sexual intercourse in the category of matters a physician might appropriately regulate—especially in the case of men. Sex, in Greek culture, reflected less the relationship between people and God (as it tended to do in Judaism and Christianity) than the hierarchies of human society, in which male citizens were on top and everyone else (boys, women, foreigners, slaves) lay beneath them. Sex, as Michel Foucault and other students of classical culture have argued, was less something that transpired *between* two people than something a man performed *on* those below him in society.[5] For a Greek physician to prescribe sexual intercourse to a free, male, adult patient was not a moral issue in a culture organized along these lines: it was simply a normal matter of bodily health. Whether the patient chose to have the sex in question with his wife, a prostitute, or a slave, or even simply to masturbate, was irrelevant.

With some adjustments, Islamic physicians had been able to maintain this principle as they perpetuated the traditions of classical medicine and science. The Islamic world was quite receptive to classical ideas—among them, Greek and Roman views on sex and disease. Though it abhorred adultery and frowned on homosexuality and masturbation, the medieval Islamic world still gave men substantial sexual liberty, permitting them to be married to as many as four women at any given time, and even to purchase female slaves for sex. "Women are replaceable!" one Islamic sage cheerfully remarked.[6]

Christian Europeans, however, saw this picture in a very different light. Filtering a Platonic idea through the Hellenistic culture of the Mediterranean world, many early Christians viewed the body as a problematic and ultimately disposable container for the eternal treasure it contained. The body was "the prison of the soul." As the great integrator and popularizer St. Paul (born Saul of Tarsus, ca. 10–ca. 67 A.D.) put it, in a formulation that ran like an electrical current through much of early and medieval Christianity, to be at home in the body was to be away from the Lord (2 Corinthians 5:8).

These views contributed to deeply ambivalent Christian attitudes toward both health and sex. Positive views of the body and its well-being were closely tied to Christ himself, who had been seen as the sacred Word made flesh, and who had made his godhead known by restoring the sick to health with miraculous cures. Indeed, as medical historian Vivian Nutton writes, Christianity has always been "a healing religion *par excellence*."[7] At the same time, however, Christianity's emphasis on the world to come meant that earthly life would ultimately be left behind. Some early Christians, therefore, argued that their fellows should joyfully welcome disaster and disease: physical suffering, they believed, led to spiritual maturity, and bodily afflictions were, as medical historians Darrel Amundsen and Gary Ferngren have observed, "designed by God to weaken the ties of the Christian to the ephemeral lures of this world."[8] Sickness and death could be accepted and even welcomed by those who viewed them as divine correctives, reminders of spiritual priorities, and ways to escape the sufferings of earthly life and enter into the kingdom of God.

Attitudes toward sex reflected a similar division. Some authorities in the early Church had positive, or at least neutral, views of sexuality. Tertullian (ca. 155–after 220), a theological moralist, believed that Christ had abolished not the sinful flesh itself, but only the sin that was *in* the flesh. St. Ambrose (ca. 340–397, bishop of Milan) agreed: "The senses themselves are only evil," he wrote, "when they are directed by an evil heart."[9] A few churchmen warmly embraced the principle of fleshly intercourse, such as St. Gregory of Nyssa (ca. 330–ca. 395), whose brother St. Basil would become famous for his gentle and generous care of the sick. The eminent historian of late antiquity Peter Brown explains that Gregory, a married bishop, believed sexuality to be "a privileged sign of God's abiding care. For God had foreseen that Adam would have need of it: in that sense, He had created human nature both in His own image, and also as male and female." Others, less enthusiastic than Gregory, accepted sex and marriage because they doubted that the Christian clergy *could* give them up. And still others, like the presbyter Clement of Alexandria (ca. 150–ca. 215), thought the whole matter was completely overblown. Clement mocked those of his peers who thought that being celibate would guarantee them salvation: "They set their hopes," he snorted, "on their private parts."

But those who tolerated sex were increasingly inundated by the pro-celibacy tide that swept over the age. Christ himself had held up celibacy as an ideal: after the Resurrection, he affirmed, "men and women do not marry: no, they are like the angels in heaven" (Matthew 22:30–31). Paul, too, had seen marriage only as a second-best alternative to virginity, a device created to help the feeble avoid the devil's constant tempting to the mortal sin of fornication. "If they cannot contain, let them marry," he wrote cheerlessly in 1 Corinthians 7, since "it is better to marry than to burn." Many of the Fathers of the Church—Origen (ca. 185–ca. 254), John Chrysostom (ca. 347–407, Patriarch of Antioch), and Augustine of Hippo (354–430)—also looked askance at sex.

As early as the second century, a powerful idea had begun to blossom among Christians: that celibacy, if widely embraced, would hasten the arrival of God's kingdom by bringing the temporal world to a rapid close. As Peter Brown explains, early Christians were convinced that

> by renouncing all sexual activity the human body could join in Christ's victory: it could turn back the inexorable [and] wrench itself free from the grip of the animal world. By refusing to act upon the youthful stirrings of desire, Christians could bring marriage and childbirth to an end. With marriage at an end, the huge fabric of organized society would crumble like a sandcastle, touched by the 'ocean flood of the Messiah.'

Sex was tied to everything these Christians wanted to escape—the body, suffering, the endless cycle of birth and death. By turning away from sex, Christians could free the world from suffering and bring heaven closer to the here and now.

With this powerful procelibacy tradition behind them, medieval

Christians were unlikely to take readily to the idea that physicians could prescribe sex freely. Resolving humoral problems was all very well, but for Christians there was a moral law that rose far above the petty importance of human plumbing. Bodily pressures could build and build, even to the point of putting life at risk; the moral laws still held. Sexual intercourse was not an activity like eating, drinking, sleeping, or exercise, to be indulged in simply because it felt good or might be considered good for the body. Sex was permissible on limited occasions and under tightly controlled circumstances. Outside of wedlock, however, sex was intolerable; a cure that healed the body and ruined the soul was worse than useless: it was anathema. Thus, lovesickness and the coital cure set up a struggle between pagan medicine and Christian morality in medieval Europe.

How did this struggle play itself out in European culture? It is exceptionally difficult to answer this question with any degree of precision: there were no demographers, no statisticians, no epidemiologists for this disease. What is known about medieval lovesickness comes from books written with certain kinds of built-in bias. Much of the story is told by medical school textbooks, which were an important source of knowledge but were also tightly bound by tradition and convention. Medieval medical writers were far more likely to repeat what their sources had written than to introduce new evidence based on what they saw in their clinics. Some books of sermons, theology, and religious stories also discussed lovesickness, but these too had an axe to grind: religious writers wanted to point their readers toward salvation. Even if these accounts are slanted, however, they show how the strange disease of lovesickness served as an early scene of conflict between two very different views of health and sex. In this battle the priorities and values of both sides emerged: some warriors placed their sights on salvation, while others cared primarily about health. And sex, as it so often would be in the following centuries, was the territory contested by the fighting sides.

GREEKS, ROMANS, AND ARABS

The idea that love could be an illness and sex a cure sounds so strange to modern ears that it is tempting to dismiss those who believed in it as medical oddballs or quacks. Little, however, could be further from the truth: the idea of lovesickness was at the center of a highly erudite and deeply respected tradition. The balance of the humors, of course, was the foundation on which the whole edifice of classical medicine was constructed, and Aristotle (384–322 B.C.) had laid additional ground-work for the theory of lovesickness by stating, in *The Generation of Animals*, that blood in both men and women could be converted into seed. (Until the discovery of spermatozoa in 1677, many doctors believed that both men and women had seed that united to give rise to the fetus.) The idea that love could cause illness had been tossed around by a number of classical poets, including the scientific Roman writer Lucretius (first century B.C.) and Ovid (43 B.C.–17 A.D.), the author of the mock-didactic treatises *The Art of Love* and *Cures for Love*, which were read widely and sometimes literally in the Middle Ages.

But it was the Greek Claudius Galen (129–199 A.D., personal physician to the Roman emperor Commodus) who gave both disease and cure the official imprimatur of the medical establishment. Often considered the most eminent physician of antiquity, Galen wrote an astounding 180 medical treatises; the fact that nearly 120 of these survive eighteen centuries later is testimony to the frequency with which his manuscripts were copied and read. When Galen diagnosed lovesickness in *On the Affected Parts*, and endorsed sexual intercourse as part of a correct regimen ("health-conscious gentlemen," he wrote, made love "even when the act gave them no particular pleasure"[10]), he virtually assured that the disease would remain on the medical books for the next sixteen hundred years.

Galen's advice on this topic, as on many others, was quoted, expounded upon, and amplified by a rapidly broadening stream of medical authorities. This scholarly torrent was virtually undiverted by the rapids of political and social change that lay between the classical period and late antiquity, and took that culture's learning over enormous cultural cascades into the Islamic and, later, medieval European worlds. One after another, almost all the great medical writers of late antiquity and the Islamic Middle Ages recommended sex as therapy for lovesickness and the larger disease from which it was derived, melancholia. One was the great Oribasius (326–403), who counted the emperor Julian the Apostate among his patients. Another was the last of the antique medical textbook authors, Paul of Aegina (ca. 625–ca. 690)—revered by the Arabs as the best Greek medical writer. "From sexual enjoyments," wrote Paul in his *Seven Books of Medicine*, "the following advantages may be derived. They relieve plethora [excess of blood], render the body lighter, promote its growth, and make it more masculine. They free the mind from the cares which beset it, and relieve it from ungovernable anger. Wherefore," he concluded, "the best possible remedy for melancholy is coition."

Oribasius and Paul were trying to maintain the Greek culture that had existed for centuries around the Mediterranean, but they lived in a time of massive social upheaval. The ancient world's greatest library, at Alexandria, was destroyed in civil wars in the late third century A.D., and a subsidiary library was burned by Christians a century later. In Europe, the fire of classical culture sank to embers that burned only in a few isolated monasteries in Ireland, Scotland, and the Swiss Alps. Mohammed (570–632) and his successors conquered the eastern Mediterranean and northern Africa in a wave of bloody wars, converting nations to the new religion of Islam. Even amidst this uproar, however, the transmission of medical knowledge continued among the Arabic-speaking peoples, as the tradition passed from book to book, language to language, sage to sage.

Almost all the great scholars of the Islamic medical world carried forward the tradition of lovesickness and its sexual cure. Among them was the eminent Avicenna, whose million-word *Canon of Medicine* remained in use in the great European medical schools of Montpellier and Louvain until 1650, and in India until after 1900.[11] Avicenna wrote of the toxic nature of pent-up sperm and the benefits of sexual intercourse as cure; if marriage was impossible, he advised, doctors should purchase female slaves and force their lovesick patients to have sex with them.[12] Therapeutic intercourse was recommended with equal enthusiasm by Rhazes, by Costa ben Luca (Qustā ibn Lūqā, 864–923), by the great synthesizer of theory and practice Haly Abbas ('Ali ibn al-'Abbās al-Magūsī, d. ca. 944), and by Abulcasis (Abu-al-Qasim Khalaf ibn-Abbas al-Zahrawi, ca. 936–ca. 1013), a physician in Moslem Spain much admired by Christian Europeans.[13]

ACROSS THE MEDITERRANEAN

Throughout the early Middle Ages, literature in Greek and Arabic remained virtually inaccessible to medieval Europeans, who had neither the books nor the linguistic skills to read them. All this began to change in the late eleventh century, however, when a shadowy figure named Constantine the African appeared on Italian shores. Medieval legends provided varying stories about Constantine's early life. One held that he had been born in Carthage and traveled throughout the Eastern world, learning all the arcane arts and sciences of Babylon, Persia, India, Ethiopia, and Egypt, until his countrymen grew jealous of his knowledge and forced him to flee to Italy, accompanied by his manuscripts. Another story made him a philanthropic merchant who, seeing a tremendous need and opportunity in Europe's lack of medical knowledge, sailed across the Mediterranean with a cargo full of books. However true or fanciful these legends, European historical records do confirm that Constantine came to the southern Italian monastery of Salerno, was welcomed by the abbot, converted to Christianity, and undertook a massive translation effort, providing Latin versions of many of the major works of Greek and Arabic medicine before he died.[14] These books were copied and recopied, and other translators fell to the task as Europeans rushed to mine this long-hidden vein of golden learning.

This is not to say, however, that the Church necessarily embraced the new knowledge. Often it fought against it as bitterly (if also as fruitlessly) as it fought against the acceptance of Aristotle. What need had Christians of secular medicine, after all? Christ was the only healer they needed. St. Bernard of Clairvaux (d. 1153) made this point to his monks: "It is not at all in keeping with your profession," he chastised them, "to seek for bodily medicines, and they are not really conducive to health. The use of common herbs, such as are used by the poor, can sometimes be tolerated, and such is our custom. But to buy special kinds of medicines, to seek out doctors and their nostrums, this does not become religious."[15] Did Bernard mean that secular medicine was ineffective, or simply that it was unseemly for monks, who should have been focused on the spirit rather than the body? It is difficult to be sure, but what is quite clear is that Bernard, like many other medieval theologians, was deeply suspicious of the medical profession and would no doubt have concurred with a cynical proverb of the day: "Out of every three physicians, two are atheists." A sermon by the thirteenth-century preacher Jacques de Vitry highlighted the struggle between medical and Christian advice. "God says 'keep vigils,'" Jacques warned his flock; but "the doctors say 'go to sleep.' God says 'fast'; the doctors say 'eat.' God says 'mortify the flesh'; the doctors say 'be comfortable.'"[16] It was not hard to tell which was the road to heaven and which to hell. Many people followed his advice, seeking cures not from greedy and sacrilegious doctors but from Christ and the saints. One modern historian estimates that 90 percent of the miracles commemorated at English and Continental shrines between 1100 and 1400 involved the healing and cure of physical ills.[17]

The conflict between medical and religious advice would come to a head when the concept of lovesickness arrived in Europe, brought by Constantine in his precious cargo of manuscripts. As Constantine translated these Arabic writings into Latin, he discussed the concept of lovesickness and the coital cure in several books—his *Medical Handbook for Travelers*, his treatise *On Melancholia*, and his aptly titled *On Sexual Intercourse*, a work so widely known that three centuries after it was written Chaucer could refer to it as a commonplace in *The Canterbury Tales*.

Quite a number of European medical authorities passed this new knowledge along to their students and readers, apparently without undue concern for the moral problems it raised. The German abbess, author, visionary, and composer Hildegard of Bingen (1098–1179) subscribed fully to the classical theory. Lovesick men, Hildegard explained in her book *Causes and Cures of Diseases*, became almost inhuman. Their faces grew dark, their eyes fiery and viperish; their veins—full of thick, black blood—grew hard. Such men were prone to madness and lust, she wrote, and rutted with women "like donkeys." Only one thing could cure them: sexual intercourse. "When they exercise their lust by overcoming women," the abbess confided, "they no longer suffer mental illness." Any problematic moral implications of this remedy, however, went unaddressed by the learned German nun.

Other medieval medical writers, more in the mainstream than the brilliant but eccentric Hildegard, also recommended sex as a cure. These included William of Saliceto (1210–1277), a professor at the universities of Bologna, Verona, Pavia, and Piacenza; Montpellier professors Arnald of Villanova (1235–1312) and Bernard of Gordon, as well as John of Gaddesden (ca. 1280–1360), an Oxford M.D. who served on the faculty of the university's Merton College. Sex was certainly not the only cure these physicians could recommend for lovesickness. Following a long tradition, they also proposed a variety of herbal medicines that ranged from the gentle to the poisonous, including thyme, pepper, pine, iris root, and myrrh, oil of violets and of roses, and the juices of mallow and sage, as well as wormwood, bitter almonds, and hellebore.[18]

In addition, they proposed psychological treatments for the disease. Some of these were pleasant measures certain to comfort and reassure the lover's melancholic mind; lovesick patients, their doctors told them, could relax in the bath, listen to music, talk with friends, recite poetry, and go for walks in verdant regions of the countryside where running streams babbled reassuringly. But just as fragrant sage and thyme were backed up by noxious hellebore and bitter wormwood, these mild and relaxing psychological expedients had darker alternatives, the medieval equivalents of aversion therapy. Some of these were merely verbal—scoldings, reproaches, and so on—but difficult cases were handled more harshly. Bernard of Gordon, for example, recommended that an authority figure counsel the lovesick patient that lust and desire placed his soul in danger of eternal torment. If this warning failed, however, Bernard noted in his *Lily of Medicine*, the patient must be beaten "until he begins to rot." Arnald of Villanova concurred with this severe treatment, advising physicians to threaten their most recalcitrant patients with castration[19]—a procedure that would be used for certain sexual problems into the Victorian era, and even beyond. (In a bizarre incident in 1999, a man in Indiana pled guilty to castrating men who wanted to curb their sexual desires. Edward Bodkin was sentenced to eighteen months in jail for practicing medicine without a license, even though he insisted that he had performed the operations "to absolve emotional, psychological, or physical needs . . . and not merely [to cater to] the spurious fancy of some alternate lifestyle." Bodkin kept several videotapes of the operations in a rented storage locker; nine jars of preserved testicles were found in his apartment.)[20]

Moral suasion and threats of violence were not the only strings on Bernard's psychological bow. Following another tradition that dated back to Ovid's first-century poem *Cures for Love*, Bernard recommended transforming passion into disgust. Ovid had offered other ruses for those wishing to fall out of love: inducing a frog-voiced girlfriend to sing; making a beloved with bad teeth laugh uproariously; visiting the object of one's unrequited affections before her makeup job was complete; and picking a posture for sex that showed off whatever blemishes one's girlfriend's figure might have. "Far be it from me," Ovid even whispered, insidiously, "to suggest that you catch a glimpse of her while she is relieving herself on the commode. . . ." Ovid hardly meant his advice to be taken seriously by his readers, but many of them failed to catch his humor. The emperor Augustus exiled the urbane poet to the barbarous shores of the Black Sea for being a bad moral influence on Roman society, and Ovid's poetic works on love, by a curious twist of fate, became primers in medieval church schools, and were regularly cited in all apparent seriousness by medieval medical writers, as well.[21]

Bernard followed Ovid's lead in the attempt to cure forlorn lovers by disgust. But the classical poet's balanced wit, which had armed both men and women for the battle of love, turned, in Bernard's less skillful hands, into a virulent misogyny. Describing a scene like something out of a lowbrow Roman comedy, Bernard suggested that old women be hired by the physician to exaggerate—and, if need be, invent—appalling defects in the face and character of the sick man's elusive beloved. They should tell the patient, said Bernard, that the reluctant mistress "is a drunkard, that she urinates in bed, that she is subject to fits, that she is a slut, that there are enormous growths on her body, and that she has bad breath." Should even these slanders fail to change the lover's deluded mind, the last resort was a visual—and olfactory—aid. The old woman should "suddenly put a used menstrual rag in front of his face, and, while holding it there, shout at him, 'This is your girlfriend— this!'"[22] Particularly in the Middle Ages, when women were blamed for Adam's fall and all the evils of human sexual nature, it was hardly surprising that falling obsessively in love was seen as a grave mental disorder and doctored with the most offensive treatments possible.

SEXUAL POLITICS AND THE WANDERING WOMB

Sexual politics, in fact, were a huge component of medical views on lovesickness. Myths, legends, and fears about women's sexuality ran freely through all parts of life in the ancient and medieval worlds, and many of them came to the fore when physicians and theologians discussed a kind of love that was already classified as a disease. This medical problem, which affected an area already taboo, clearly put doctors in an extremely awkward position—and this position revealed much about how medieval society looked at the tangled relationship of sex with disease and sin.

Medieval doctors were hardly the first to tremble with anxiety about women's bodies and their obscure needs. Classical scientists and physicians had seen women as cold, moist creatures whose clammy humors threatened to extinguish the dry heat that burned in men; some even believed that women's bodies held a deadly poison.[23] Furthermore, females were viewed as sexually insatiable: "the more women have sex, the more they desire it," warned Gerard de Solo (ca. 1305–late fourteenth century), chancellor of the University of Montpellier.[24]

The organ that symbolized all these fears was the womb. This most female part of the body was called the *hystera* in Greek, and as far back as in ancient Egypt, the womb had been associated with the complex psychosomatic illness that came to be known as hysteria. In addition— perhaps because the womb sometimes became prolapsed, descending downward into the vagina, or even outside it—people believed that it could roam freely around the body. Plato (427?–347 B.C.), for example, called it "an animal within an animal," an unattached organ with a mind and will of its own. "The womb is an animal that longs to generate children," the philosopher taught. "When it remains barren long after puberty, it is distressed and sorely disturbed. Straying about in the body and cutting off the passages of the breath, it impedes respiration and brings the sufferer into extremest anguish and provokes all manner of diseases besides. . . . Such is the nature of women and all that is female."[25]

The unsatisfied womb, yearning for the delights of sex and fertility, did everything it could to control the woman whose body it inhabited. The second-century A.D. medical writer Aretaeus of Cappadocia, for example, explained all the dreadful symptoms of the "hysterical" condition, and advised proper treatment for the woman so affected. A wandering uterus, he explained, could travel far enough up the woman's inner cavity to strangle her, cutting off her breathing so quickly that she would not even have a moment to cry out for help. The physician must rush to the aid of the unconscious patient, Aretaeus counseled, cutting open the veins at her ankles so excess blood could flow out, and tying her hands and feet so that no involuntary motion was possible. Then he should use the subterfuge of odor to trick the troublesome organ to return to its proper place. At the woman's nose, the doctor must put evil-smelling substances such as old urine, burnt hair, and pitch, to drive her womb away from the respiratory organs, while, at her genitals, cinnamon and other delightful fragrances should be placed to lure it back down. Once it had redescended, the uterus must be trapped in place, compressed by the hands of "a strong woman or an expert man" and "bound around with a roller so it would not escape." Then, finally, the doctor should rouse the unconscious patient by bathing her body, rubbing her face, and plucking out her hair.

Galen dismissed the wandering uterus as a myth, but he firmly believed that the lack of sex caused endless troubles for women. It could make them hysterical; it could cause them to retain their menses; and it could be responsible for a buildup of semen, just as it was in lovesick men. Particularly for widows, who had been accustomed to the joys of intercourse and the satisfactions of fertility, "the female semen is a burden."[26] Stool, urine, semen, menses—all must be voided on a regular basis, Galen advised.

The problem with this theory, of course, was that neither in Greece or Rome, nor in the worlds of medieval Islam and Christianity, did women have the kind of sexual freedom men enjoyed. The fact that women might *need* sex did not mean that they were allowed to *have* it. As a result, physicians tried to find ways to keep their female patients healthy without breaking what they saw as the laws of morality, society, and nature. Arabic-language medical authorities such as Rhazes, Haly Abbas, Avicenna, and Abulcasis suggested that women troubled by a buildup of menses or semen could be treated with vaginal fumigations or with massage; sometimes these doctors would go so far as to suggest that the mouth of the uterus could be stimulated by a midwife who had lubricated her fingers with fragrant oils, releasing the woman's seed in paroxysms of female pleasure.

On female troubles, European physicians were generally even more cautious than their Islamic counterparts. Herbs, medicinal diets, and fumigations they could certainly countenance, but any smell of sex— even the slightest whiff—set off moral alarms. William of Saliceto, for example, knew his medical textbooks well. He understood that the lack of sex put women in danger; he knew that stimulation could clear up the problem; and he was willing to violate some rules of propriety by having the midwife rub the opening of the sick woman's vulva "hard." But that was as far as he was willing to go. "If she is married," he advised, "let her use sexual intercourse. If she is not yet married, let her marry. And if she does not yet wish to marry, let her be cured by bloodlettings and purges with foul-smelling pills and such."[27] Doctors could prescribe the healthful pleasures of sex if the patient had a husband. For single women, however, the only possible treatments were harsh: noxious medicines, or the sharp stab of the lancet in the vein.

INTO THEIR OWN HANDS

Unauthorized penises were clearly off limits to these women. Moral scruples hardly stopped at the phallus: anything that penetrated the woman's inner sanctum, in fact, was a grave threat to the masculine order. Even the midwife's oiled finger carried with it unsavory associations with lesbianism, and the thought of any other object exploring these forbidden recesses was so alarming that it could send tremors down the most intrepid spine.

Arnald of Villanova was a case in point. Arnald scarcely seemed the kind of person to be terrified by what later generations would refer to as a "marital aid." A brilliant, multifaceted man, Arnald lived a varied and adventuresome life: he taught at the medical school of Montpellier, served as personal physician to three kings and two popes, and carried out international diplomatic missions. He also worked to reform the Church—an effort for which he was convicted of heresy and thrown into prison. His writings spanned a rainbow of subjects (some of them quite controversial), including alchemy, magic, astrology, theology, and necromancy. These books were translated from their original Latin into many vernaculars—French, Provençal, Spanish, Italian, German, English, and even Hebrew—and more than a hundred editions of his works, printed in the fifteenth through the eighteenth centuries, still survive. A century before the Renaissance, Arnald of Villanova was a Renaissance man.

With his breadth of learning and experience, it was hardly surprising that Arnald was something of an expert on lovesickness. He mentioned it in several works, including *The Mirror of Medicine* and *The King of Aragon's Health Plan*, and even wrote a treatise devoted entirely to love. He acknowledged that sex was part of a healthy regimen, and among other less controversial cures for lovesickness, he mentioned therapeutic intercourse, if only in passing.[28] In another work, *The Practical Breviary*, he even recommended the coital cure to those suffering from "excessive abstinence," including both widows and monks. Although perhaps medically correct, from a theological point of view this was heresy plain and simple—as Arnald must have known full well.

But although Arnald had the audacity to recommend sexual intercourse to monks and was willing to go to jail for church reform, he was not made of iron, and in Florence he learned of something that shocked him to his core. Florentine women apparently suffered frequently from all the ills of sexual abstinence after they were widowed, or when their merchant husbands were away on extended business travel. Rather than rely on physicians, these resourceful women took matters into their own hands: to assuage their sexual desires, they would stimulate themselves with their fingers, or with an artificial device specifically made for this purpose—"a small stuffed bag in the shape of a man's penis." Some of the devices were far more elaborate than this, Arnald wrote in dismay. Forged in brass or bronze, these fancy dildos were hollow inside; their users filled them with rosewater, which the dildos would release just at the moment when the women released their seed. The doctor-diplomat admired the ingenuity of these objects, but he could not under any circumstances endorse their use, which, he noted, was nothing other than sodomy, the worst sexual sin of all. Instead, he recommended that women suffering from the ill effects of abstinence "have sexual intercourse with men, and so commit a lesser sin."[29]

This sounds like a practical compromise in the face of a deadly threat to health. In fact, however, Arnald was scarcely escaping from the moral dilemma, because on this point the whole tradition of Greco-Arabic medicine—the very basis of medieval medical knowledge—was at odds with the central principles of the Catholic Church. In trying to find a compromise, all Arnald could do was urge his patients to commit the sin of fornication—less horrific, perhaps, but nevertheless mortal. Lovesickness put medieval physicians into an impossible position. If their patients followed the advice of every known medical authority and practiced therapeutic intercourse, they were damned for eternity. If they did not, they were dead.

By Arnald's time, the Church had made its views on this particular topic quite clear: if Church doctrine came into conflict with medical tradition, the latter was consigned to the dunghill. In any conflict between body and soul, the soul came first. The Church repeatedly announced that neither doctors nor patients had the right even to discuss sex as therapy, and it was perfectly willing to see people die if they had to. What was the point in saving the temporal body, if in the process a patient lost his or her immortal soul? Cure or no cure, sex out of wedlock was fornication, and at that point all discussion stopped.

THE DEADLY SIN OF DEPRESSION

What looked like a medical problem to medieval physicians often seemed like a moral issue to the medieval Church. The Church believed that hysteria was caused by an alliance with "unholy powers," notes medical historian Ilza Veith, and "dejection" was seen as dangerously antisocial behavior. An Old Irish penitential manual (ca. 800 A.D.), for example, made this quite plain. It ordered that a monk "whom the Devil has mocked by means of grief and sorrows, such as the loss of friends or relatives, so that it allows him to do nothing good, but [only] to despair," be sentenced to three days of complete fasting, deprived of all food and drink. A relapse would earn the despondent monk forty days on bread and water alone, and "if he should be in grief or sadness so that he cannot be roused," he should be separated from the community and do penance on this spartan diet, not returning "until he be joyful in body and soul."[30]

This striking example shows how far Church thinking could be from that of medieval (and modern) medicine. Physicians saw melancholia as a disease, one closely related to what we now call depression, and they tried to treat the mind by easing the body. (Greek medicine, from its earliest beginnings, had treated mental problems as closely linked to physical disorders.) But for churchmen, these mental troubles were a different kind of threat. At the least, they revealed a disordered attitude; at the worst, they were a mortal sin. All human ills came from man's wicked nature, and had to be harshly punished so that the evil could be torn up by its roots.

The link between melancholy and sin was clearly explained in the *Dialogue of Miracles*, an immensely popular book of religious stories written by the German monk Caesarius of Heisterbach (ca. 1170–ca. 1240). For Caesarius, melancholy was one of the seven deadly sins— *accedia*, or sloth. *Accedia*, Caesarius explained, "is a depression born from a troubled mind, or a sense of weariness or bitterness of heart, by which spiritual happiness is cast out, and the judgment is overthrown by a headlong fall into despair." This sin gave rise to many "daughters," warned Caesarius—among them, "malice, rancor, cowardice, despair, reluctance to obey, and the straying of thoughts into forbidden places." The passions of resentment, insubordination, and illicit desire all grew from this blackened, sinful root, as Caesarius showed in his holy stories. Victims of *accedia* he catalogued included a nun, weak in faith, who threw herself into the Moselle; a young man so addicted to gambling that he bet away his own clothes and then committed suicide; and a young girl abandoned by her lover who hanged herself in despair. These case histories, for the monastic author, were not people in need of medical help, but moral outcasts in whose sinful footsteps good Christians must fear to tread. (Contemporary debates on needle exchange for drug addicts reflect some of the same dynamics.) No wonder, then, that the newly arrived concept of lovesickness—a disease born of one mortal sin and cured by another—alarmed the thirteenth-century Church.

This, at least, is what the most orthodox churchmen believed, and often their views prevailed. In 1215, for example, the Fourth Lateran Council expressly prohibited medical treatment by sinful means—specifically including sex outside of marriage. Fornication was evil, intoned William of Auvergne (bishop of Paris 1228–1249), reminding his flock of Paul's dictum that it was better to marry than to burn. Fornication was a crime, warned Bishop Bartholomew of Exeter. It was a mortal sin, declared the theologian William of Auxerre (ca. 1150–1230), and any arguments to the contrary, thundered Etienne Tempier, bishop of Paris in 1270, were heretical.[31] Doctors were not to prescribe fornication or masturbation to their patients, the Lateran Council ordered; if they did, patients were under orders to disobey.[32] Not all ecclesiastics and Catholic doctors were as orthodox as they were supposed to be, and those who were not had reason to worry: as late as the seventeenth century, one physician who recommended therapeutic intercourse was burned at the stake. For him, at least, lovesickness clearly *was* a fatal disease.

Lovesickness was part of a profound struggle within the Church, which spent much of the later Middle Ages trying to come to terms with the new learning that had arrived from the classical and Islamic worlds. Could there be a balance between Aristotle and Augustine?

Was theology still queen of the sciences, as the conservative theologians of the Sorbonne insisted? Was sex outside of marriage so incontrovertibly evil that it could not be used to save a life? These were major moral controversies in the thirteenth century, and the struggle was played out in classrooms, consulting rooms, and confessionals.

THE SIN OF LUST

Certainly there was a very strong presumption that sex was bad. Even within marriage, sex was suspect—largely because it felt good. For medieval Christians, explains legal historian James Brundage, "marital sex was free from sin as long as no one enjoyed it." Outside of marriage, of course, having sex was one of the gravest sins a Christian could commit—as evil as perjury, or even murder, wrote Gratian, the foremost canon lawyer of the Middle Ages. Two other twelfth-century authorities, Albert of Aachen and Guibert of Nogent, agreed. Just like later writers who would argue that sexually transmitted diseases came as divine retribution for sinful behavior, these medieval churchmen firmly believed that "God was perfectly capable of reaching out and exacting terrible retribution from the sexual offender in this life as well as in the next."[33] Nothing was too fearsome to be attributed to sexual sin.

It is important not to forget that the people making these savage declarations had their own struggles with the Church's sexual laws. In the earliest years, Christian clergy had been allowed to marry, but the push for clerical celibacy began in the fourth century and grew stronger and stronger over time; by 1059, marriage was formally forbidden to Christian clerics. Priests hated these new rules; some of them even stoned and burned to death Church officials who ordered them to give up their wives. Lay people often liked the new strictures no better. After all, as a contemporary chronicler cited by Brundage reported, the people were quite convinced that "a priest can not live alone, and therefore it is better that he have his own wife, for otherwise he will pursue everybody else's wives and sleep with them."[34]

If the promarriage crowd enforced its views with fire and stone, those promoting celibacy were equally severe. St. Birgitta of Sweden (1303–1373), for example, said that any pope who permitted priests to marry should have his eyes plucked out, his tongue, lips, nose, ears, hands, and feet hacked away, and all the blood drained out of his body until his cold corpse was thrown to wild beasts to devour—spiritually speaking, of course.[35]

In this moral climate, the concept of coitus as therapy provoked

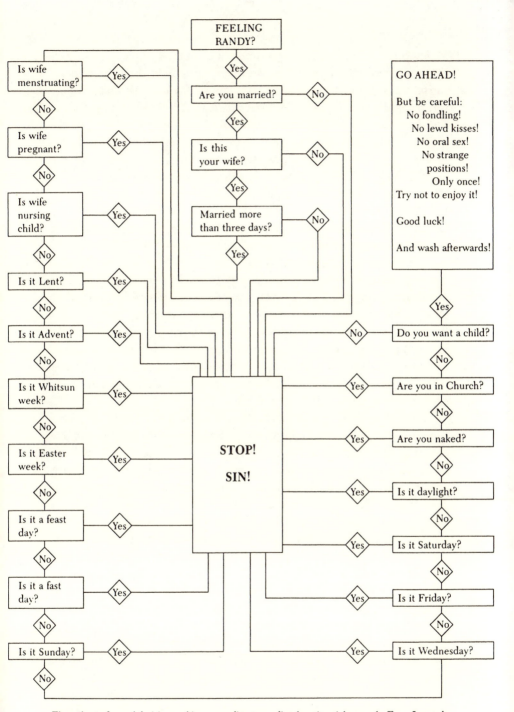

Flow-chart of sexual decision making, according to medieval penitential manuals. From James A. Brundage, *Law, Sex, and Christian Society in Medieval Europe* (Chicago: University of Chicago Press, 1984).

strong opposition, and this opposition was only reinforced by the fact that the problem was attracting so much notice. At least three major thirteenth-century theologians—William of Auxerre, William of Auvergne, and Bishop Vincent of Beauvais (ca. 1190–1264, author of the *Speculum quadruplex* [The four-way mirror], perhaps the greatest medieval encyclopedia)—talked about lovesickness, and acknowledged how serious an affliction it was. But recognizing the problem was not the same thing as solving it, particularly when the cure was so controversial. William of Auxerre, attempting to mold Greek science to Christian doctrine, announced timidly that "this disease has its cure in medicine and diet."[36] The two bishops, however, while fretting about the problem ("a most serious mental alienation," admitted William of Auvergne) failed to mention a single remedy.[37]

Such ambiguities were good enough for academic theologians, but more popular writers took a much harder line: in story after story, they showed their readers what was right and what was wrong. These colorful cases give a valuable insight into the way lovesickness made its way into the popular culture of the age, and show what people were taught to believe. Time after time, these examples rammed home the message that lust was a sin, and that cures for this and for all bodily afflictions came directly—and only—from Christ.

Some of these stories dated back to the fathers of the Church: St. Gregory (ca. 540–604), for example, told an edifying tale about the purity of St. Benedict (480–543). Trying to cleanse his soul in the wilderness, Benedict was tormented by the devil, who filled his head with images of a woman he desired. Do what he might, the saint could not get her out of his mind, and was almost at the point of abandoning his quest for virtue in order to satisfy his lust. Finally, however, God came to his aid: divine grace led Benedict to a thicket of briars and nettles. The holy man stripped off his clothes and plunged in, and the stings and lacerations he experienced conquered once and for all the inner prickings of his lust. "From that time forward," Benedict announced to his approving followers, "he found all temptation of pleasure so subdued that he never more felt any such thing."[38]

Caesarius of Heisterbach told many stories about how to deal with lust. Each in its own way taught that the body and its longings were vile, and that Christians were happiest when they left these burdens behind. Some of these stories were simply odd, like that of the nun who conquered temptation by banging her head against a door, or another who was saved from illicit love by a box on the ear given by the Blessed Virgin herself. Others, however, had a more melancholy and disturbing

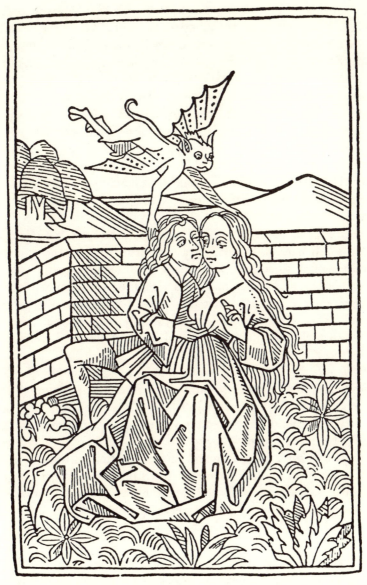

Thou Shalt Not Commit Adultery: The Evil Spirit Presides over the Embraces of Lovers. Woodcut from the Augsburg *Ten Commandments* (1478).

tinge. One nun, for example, fell in love with the man who was the head of her convent; her desire burned and burned until the day when she finally confessed her desires to her beloved. Without uttering a word, the man stripped off his outer garments and the hair shirt he wore beneath them to torment his flesh. He "showed her his naked body, eaten with vermin, scarred with the hair shirt, and black with grime," and then announced, "See what it is that you love, and take your pleasure if you still desire it." Needless to say, the nun's desire instantly vanished. In another story, a knight's incestuous desire to marry his cousin was immediately removed when he took communion from St. Bernard of Clairvaux. That he died immediately thereafter in no way diminished the success of the cure—at least as far as Caesarius was concerned.

Given such views of lust, the Church's hard-line stance on lovesickness was only natural. Indeed, it was surprising that any theologians at all were willing to see the disease as a medical problem that doctors should address, and that some should accept sex as a legitimate remedy (though only, of course, when the sexual partner was the patient's spouse).[39] But when the spouse was not within reach, or when there was no spouse at all, then the higher moral standard prevailed, as two final stories show.

The Jewel of the Church, a book of popular piety written by Gerald of Wales (1146?–1223?) told the stories of two eminent victims of lovesickness whose differing fates pointed a single moral. One, King Louis VII of France, fell ill in Burgundy while engaged in a military campaign. The queen was too far away to reach him in time, and doctors proposed that some other woman be found to offer her body to restore the king's health; the bishops even assured their royal leader that they would clear his actions with God. Louis, however, had no patience for such theological quackery. If no other cure could be found, he proudly announced, "then I choose rather to die a chaste man than live an adulterer."

A bishop of Louvain fell ill with the same complaint. Abstinence swelled his genitals to huge proportions; his life was in mortal danger. "Take a woman!" urged the ever-present counselors. Like King Louis, however, the afflicted bishop held fast to his virtue. "I will by no means for the sake of my temporal life," he swore, "bring shame to my sacred order, my honor and dignity, and damage to my soul by doing what you suggest. I may die in my body," he piously concluded, "but through God's grace I will live in eternal life."

Two lives hung in the balance. What happened? One was spared, and one was lost. God saved Louis, explained Gerald, for the good of France: he needed the king to win battles for his people and to beget an heir. The bishop, on the other hand, served God better dead. His life had been a shining example of piety, and his sainted corpse performed miracles for the faithful. What was most important about these two stories, Gerald explained, was that they taught a single lesson. What mattered was not these men's earthly lives, but their obedience to God's will.

Only with the Permission of Faith and Law

This is why Church writers could not mention therapeutic intercourse. Of course it made sense in terms of Greek medicine; but to the Greeks, the body had been primarily a physical object, akin in nature to a machine. Christians, however, had to think not just about the paltry threescore years and ten the Bible allotted to one's earthly existence—a figure that was typically cut in half in the European Middle Ages, when disease, malnutrition, catastrophic weather, and wars were as common as rats and fleas. There was the starkness of eternity to consider, and in the face of endless eons of heavenly bliss or diabolical torment, even a life-threatening illness scarcely mattered.

This doctrine was severely maintained for centuries. Lovesickness continued to appear in medical books into the 1600s and 1700s, and the Church's formal position on it did not moderate, as one seventeenth-century Italian doctor, Giulio Cesare Vanini, learned at the cost of his life. Vanini endorsed sexual intercourse as a cure, and this lapse and others (he had also attacked Church doctrine and approved of medical astrology) provoked the authorities to condemn him to strangling by the iron collar of the garotte, after which he was burned at the stake for good measure.

Vanini's contemporary Jacques Ferrand was wise enough to take warning from his colleague's untimely end. The first edition of Ferrand's treatise on lovesickness (1645) discussed the forbidden remedy, and as a direct result of this transgression, both the Church and the Parliament of Toulouse ordered that the book be burned. A later version showed that Dr. Ferrand had learned how to be prudent: discussing therapeutic intercourse: he cautioned in the second edition that there was an enormous distinction between "licit and illicit lovemaking." Marriage made the cure acceptable, of course. "But if for any reason a marriage cannot be contracted," warned the chastened author, "it is totally absurd and immoral to prescribe, as Avicenna and Haly Abbas do, that our lover 'purchase young girls and sleep with them frequently, and that he change them regularly and take his pleasure with new ones.'" Presumably Ferrand had realized that burning at the stake was far more painful—and far more deadly—than burning with lust.[40]

The story of lovesickness in the Middle Ages shows how high the stakes could be in the battle over bodies and souls. Each side of the debate had the weight of tradition and authority behind it: the Church, of course, had the Bible, the Fathers, and centuries of sacred doctrine on its side, all testifying to the moral frailty of the body, beset on every side by temptation and sin. Disease, in this tradition, was ultimately a symptom of humanity's wicked nature, and the only true and sure remedies were those provided by the Redeemer. The medical tradition had its own saints—Hippocrates, Galen, the late antique compilers, and the shining intellectual lights of the medieval Arabic-speaking world—and its own sacred traditions, including the fundamental principles of humoral medicine and the belief that it was a doctor's duty to regulate such matters as food and sexual intercourse to preserve a patient's health. Neither of these ancient and authoritative views of the body totally denied the other's point of view. Some churchmen acknowledged that academic medicine had much to offer, even in the vexed case of lovesickness; some physicians—Avicenna among them—acknowledged that the sexual remedy should be prescribed only "with the permission of faith and law."

But in many ways lovesickness pushed the differences to the limits. When a patient was dying, and only a sinful cure was available, what was the doctor to do, and what could the priest advise? Each stared hard at the other, and someone had to blink. Cases came to different conclusions, as our stories have shown: sometimes medicine yielded, sometimes faith. Often, probably, it was the patient who ultimately gave way. But regardless of the individual outcomes, what remained was a sharp cultural divide between those who worried mostly about the body and those whose greatest concern was the soul. This fissure was to underlie every case of sex and disease that was to follow lovesickness—from leprosy to syphilis, and, ultimately, all the way to AIDS.

CHAPTER TWO

To Live Outside the Camp: Medieval Leprosy

While academic physicians and theologians were disputing the finer points of lovesickness, most ordinary people in the European Middle Ages had far more urgent trials to worry them. Their bodies were racked by famine, riven by wars, and assaulted by extreme weather and the onslaught of disease after disease. "Death was omnipresent," writes historian D. H. Pennington, "and witnessing it was everyone's experience."[1] Beyond the ever-present reality of malnutrition, people suffered from many diseases, including plague, fevers, scrofula, and tuberculosis. All of these were brutal, but one of the diseases they feared most was the slow and loathsome disintegration of leprosy.

Leprosy was an African disease that had become endemic in Europe by the end of the sixth century.[2] It terrified people because it was disfiguring, disgusting, and mysterious in whom it chose to afflict. Some physicians believed the disease was hereditary; others said it was spread by contagion, although scientific and medical theory could not really explain how contagion worked. Some believed that sexual intercourse transmitted or caused the hideous affliction. No matter what they thought was its source, many people believed that leprosy came straight from God to punish humanity for its sins.

This belief was so strong, and the patterns it etched so searing, that they remained deep in the European heart for centuries. A century and more after leprosy had departed from Western Europe, moldering medieval leper hospitals were reopened to serve as isolation wards for the corrupt souls and bodies of heretics and syphilitics. Decrepit, isolated, and accursed, the medieval leper remained for centuries a symbol of the worst that God could visit on humanity.

"UNCLEAN, UNCLEAN"

Spreading slowly throughout the body, the leprosy bacterium damages the nerves and keeps the blood from supplying oxygen and nutrients to the skin; secondary infections descend on dying flesh like birds of prey on carrion. First they raise unsightly calluses and scars; then fingers, toes, and sections of nasal tissue fall away. Hands and feet are twisted into bear-claw shapes; the face becomes broken and twisted; nasal cartilage and vocal cords are damaged, and the voice becomes raspy and honking. As tubercular lesions protrude, the eyebrows become swollen and denuded of hair; the face, the skin, and the limbs take on frightening new aspects; the mouth and nostrils become twisted; the eyes take on a horrifying stare; and breath and body often give off a disgusting smell.[3]

With these stark and offensive transformations, it is hardly surprising that the impulse to fear, loathe, and isolate lepers was ancient and enduring. A disease that the Middle Ages identified as leprosy had been mentioned in Leviticus 13, and the words of this Old Testament passage would resonate throughout Western history like the clappers medieval lepers were compelled to carry to warn the uninfected away. "A man afflicted with leprosy," commanded the Hebrew law, "must wear his clothing torn and his hair disordered; he must shield his upper lip and cry, 'Unclean, unclean.' As long as the disease lasts he must be unclean, and therefore he must live apart; he must live outside the camp." Despite the severity of the pronouncements, explains one scholar, lepers were not completely cut off from the Hebrew community: instead, "they were viewed as both chosen and rejected by God" and were considered a kind of living dead. Their disease—diagnosed not by doctors but by priests—was seen as a frightening but awesome mark from God.

This pattern was not universal: lepers were allowed to roam freely in Byzantium and in the medieval Islamic world. But ancient Greek historians noted that other cultures they observed would not tolerate lepers among the general population. Pausanias, in 479 B.C., recorded that a town in Elida was called Leproon because so many lepers lived there; in Persia, Herodotus (484?–425? B.C.) observed, lepers were driven from cities. The ten lepers Jesus healed in Luke 17 "stood afar off" from him while begging to be healed; the Greek doctors of the

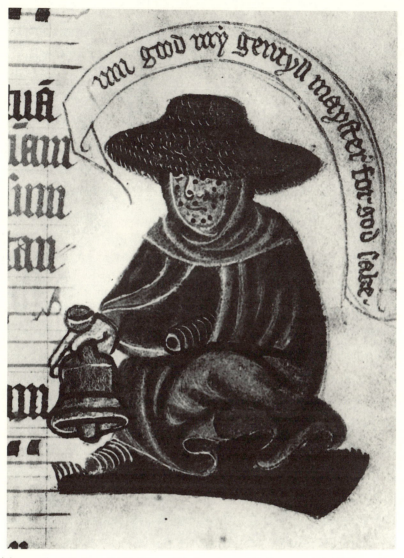

A leper with a bell. From British Library MS. Lansdowne 451. Courtesy of the Wellcome Trust Medical Photographic Library, London. "Sum good myn gentyll mayster for god sake."

sixth and seventh centuries A.D. noted that their cities drove lepers away. Some of this separation was no doubt caused simply by revulsion, and some of it may have been caused by medical fears, but in Europe, at least, the greatest concern was sin. As medical historian Katharine Park explains, medieval European laws "aimed to set lepers apart as foci of moral and ritual defilement rather than as threats to public health."[4]

The ruin leprosy inflicted on people's bodies reflected in some way God's judgment on their souls, and most people wanted to have little to do with either.

The twelfth and thirteenth centuries were the height of the disease's spread in Europe, and the laws of these years often reflected people's desire to put the safety of distance between themselves and the afflicted—especially those who were both afflicted and poor. The laws of the kingdom of Navarre in 1155 ordered those lepers who could not support themselves to "beg alms in the city, outside doors, using the noise of the clappers" alone to solicit the attention and charity of passers-by, avoiding all conversation with children and the young. The Third Lateran Council (1179) relegated lepers to "solitary places" outside the walls of cities and towns. By 1220, notes one historian, "it was a civil crime for a leper to dwell among the healthy," and in 1278 the laws of Metz set up an elaborate intelligence system for weeding out lepers, with serious penalties for those who failed to cooperate. A leper who did not turn himself in would have an ear cut off; the citizen who gave him alms was fined. Police who failed to turn lepers in were subject to severe strictures; a citizen of Calais is recorded as having been punished for sheltering his leprous brother.[5]

Cities and countries passed laws that drove the afflicted out. The twelfth-century Burrow laws and thirteenth-century Church canons expelled lepers from Scotland. Gloucester expelled lepers in 1273, London in 1276, Bristol in 1344, and Norwich in 1375; the Scots parliament in 1427 forbade lepers to beg in town. Paris banned them in 1321, 1371, 1388, 1394, 1402, and 1403—so often, in fact, that one prominent French historian suggests that the bans cannot have been very effective.[6] Effective or no, however, this insistent legislation testified to the fact that, even if lepers remained in town, they were as unwelcome as rats.

Those laws that did not send lepers out of town made certain that they were easy to spot and avoid. In some areas, lepers (like Jews) were made to wear yellow badges; in others, the markers were red. To avoid soiling even the dirt in the medieval streets—streets that often flowed with raw sewage and the blood of animals slaughtered in butchers' stalls—lepers were forced to wear shoes at all times. They had to carry a clapper or a bell to warn people to keep their distance. They could not touch items in the market; instead, they had to point them out with a long pole. Begging was a necessity for them, but it was also exceptionally difficult. Lepers had to use their poles to retrieve their begging cups from the side of the road, since they were not allowed to approach those whom they solicited for farthings and crusts of bread. The citizens of Arras, in France, made official complaints when they caught lepers handling the fruit in vendors' baskets in the town market.[7] Without being quite willing to let the diseased starve in the woods, Europeans did everything they could not to have to touch, speak with, interact with, or even see those marked by this malady of body and soul.

HOSPITALS: THE HOUSE OF GOD

Those who were more compassionate tried to find a middle way, setting up a broad array of charitable hospitals to shelter the sick. The number of these leper houses reached a high-water mark in medieval Europe, but the tradition had started far earlier. Leper hospitals, in fact, were among the earliest medical establishments in the West.

Hospitals were born from the central Christian values of charity and healing. By the third century A.D., urban Christians had organized large-scale efforts to help the poor and the sick, and in the fourth century the first Western hospital had been founded by St. Basil of Caesarea, who had studied medicine in Athens. Basil welcomed strangers, the crippled, and lepers to his care, and would greet his patients with a kiss before treating their afflictions and dressing their wounds himself. In the fourth century, a wealthy Roman noble established a hospital specifically for lepers, and the emperor Constantius soon built another.[8] This prototype gave rise to two different models. In Byzantium—and, following this model, in Islam—Basil's charity toward the sick combined with the traditions of Greek medicine, and produced hospitals primarily focused on medical care. Islamic hospitals also devoted resources to pharmacy, clinical training, mental health, and research, and, being essentially secular institutions, they were able to enhance their staffs by hiring Christian and Jewish physicians.[9]

Hospitals in Western Europe followed quite a different path. They viewed themselves essentially as religious institutions dedicated to providing charity in accordance with Christian views; medical care was only incidental to this mission. Some hospitals, for example, lodged and fed poor travelers (though only for a night or two; after that, the vagrants were sent on their way). Others took on the responsibility of keeping poor women out of the clutches of vice. Statutes were written to ensure that hospital inmates behaved properly: charity was dispensed to the poor only when they adhered to the strict laws of virtue.[10]

Gradually, hospitals became more specialized. Some focused on providing temporary shelter for the poor, while some housed and cared for the sick; in France, the latter were called Hôtels-Dieu, Houses of God. Others were specifically built to house, on a more permanent basis, those who suffered from the incurable affliction of leprosy. The earliest English leper houses were founded before 1100; in Scotland and France, the first establishments began in the twelfth century, probably in response to the increasing prevalence of the disease. Their numbers grew rapidly: by the death of the French king Louis VIII in 1226, there were 1,000 leper houses in France, and Louis IX (St. Louis, 1214–1270) founded 340 more.[11] These mostly small establishments were deliberately kept humble, and their furnishings could not fail to remind the "brothers" and "sisters" of why they were there. The regulations of the late twelfth-century English leper house of Sherburne, for example, ordered that "in the house itself, they should have four lead cisterns, four pans, four tripods, two tubs, one broom, and a spade for burying the dead." Some French leper houses were painted red to warn off unwary passers-by.[12]

Even when they were built to care for the sick, however, the primary purpose of medieval hospitals was charitable rather than medical. The Paris Hôtel-Dieu, for example, which had been founded in the seventh century, recorded no medical personnel at all from 1066 to 1154; from 1154 to 1328, physicians and surgeons dropped in only occasionally. Only after the mid-fourteenth-century did the Hôtel-Dieu and its counterparts elsewhere in France maintain a regular medical staff.[13] Even with this increased interest in caring for their inmates' ailing bodies, however, what mattered most to French hospitals were spotless morals. Arriving, patients were required to make confession; only after this were they admitted and their physical needs attended to. The sacrament was no mere formality: it was as strictly required as evidence of insurance is at any American hospital today. "No sick person shall be admitted," warned the statutes of the St.-Pol hospital, "unless he first be confessed." The rules at Gautois highlighted these requirements, and underlined them in red: "If the poor man is not willing to do this, let him be sent away."

Once admitted, patients had more rules to follow. Hospital regulations prescribed penalties for many transgressions. Theft and homicide, for example, guaranteed that inmates would be expelled. But sex raised the biggest red flag of all. The rules of the Hôtel-Dieu of Pontoise, for example, noted that sins of the flesh were "to be punished more severely than all other sins," and the Hôtel-Dieu of Vernon required its "sisters" to avoid being seen by others when they were changing clothes. These women were required to keep their robes on until they were under the

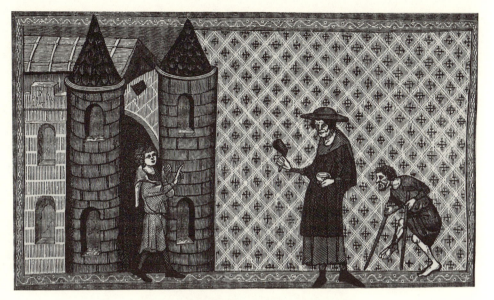

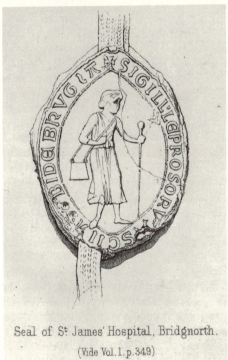

Seal of St James' Hospital, Bridgnorth.
(Vide Vol. 1. p. 349)

Thirteenth-century leper house; a leper with staff and pouch. Vincent de Beauvais, miniature, *Miroir historial*, Arsenal Library, Paris. Seal of St. James's Hospital, Bridgnorth. Courtesy of the Wellcome Trust Medical Photographic Library, London.

covers, which were to be pulled up to their breasts and kept there. (Most people in the Middle Ages slept nude.) Finally, at bedtime, these female residents were instructed to cross themselves, "in the name of the Father and the Son and the Holy Ghost, amen, against the adversities and temptations of the devil."

Those who slid beneath these moral standards were severely punished. Any sister convicted of sins of the flesh at Vernon, for example, had to do penance for forty days by lying on her back on the threshold of the chapter house, so that all the other sisters, on their way in and out, would "be able to step on her, like vileness and filth."[14] All this had little to do with health, but everything to do with virtue. Historians agree that in these hospitals, the soul came first, the body second. Admittedly, most people believed that physical and spiritual health went hand in hand. But in a narrow passageway, there was no question: religion walked first, and, if necessary, alone.[15]

EXPELLED FOREVER

If these characteristics were true of hospitals, they were doubly true of leper houses. Nobody expected lepers to recover from their condition: the leprosaria simply sheltered them until they died. As Katharine Park has crisply observed, these institutions "were charitable rather than therapeutic."[16] And charity was strictly defined: as in other hospitals, strict obedience was required in all matters. The statutes of the leper house of Amiens, dating from 1305, ordained that "if any of the brothers or sisters does anything dishonorable, he will be punished at the master's will according to the counsel of the brothers."

The lepers had considerable authority in this area, in fact. Some people came to leper houses of their own accord; others were turned in when people denounced them to the public authorities. Sometimes, parents even brought in their own children. However they came, those suspected of leprosy had to be judged by a panel of experts made up of the lepers themselves; only in the fifteenth century did doctors and surgeons join the tribunal. The judgment was taken very seriously. The men and women who served on the panel had to swear to judge accurately; if they refused to participate, they could be fined. The examinations were as scientific as the knowledge of the day permitted. There was a comprehensive visual inspection (leper houses even had a special heated room so that in winter suspects could be examined without their clothes), followed by blood and urine tests; sometimes suspects were sent to other leper houses for a second opinion. Both lepers and physicians were reluctant to misdiagnose, since, for most lepers, the sentence was irreversible.[17]

Not all lepers were able to reside in leper houses, which were usually reserved for citizens of the cities that had built them. All others—unless their families made a substantial gift to the endowment—were condemned to wander the world and beg for their sustenance. As a result, the severest punishment the administrators could impose was expulsion—cutting lepers off from food, shelter, and the only human society they were allowed to join.

Of the many things lepers could do wrong, two provoked the greatest anxiety: running away and having sex. Often, these misadventures were viewed as related: statutes forbade spending the night anywhere but under the administrators' watchful eye. For passing a night in town, Amiens would expel lepers for a year and a day, and then impose forty days' penance on them when they returned. Leper houses in the British Isles were even more severe, as historian Charles Arthur Mercier records: "At Greenside, in Scotland, the same offense was a hanging matter, and lest any leper should plead that he knew not, or had forgotten the penalty, the authorities thoughtfully set up a gibbet before the gate of the hospital to remind him."[18]

These punishments were stringent for a reason: leprosy had been associated with sin since biblical times. King Ozias, in 2 Chronicles, had been punished with leprosy for his sacrilege; the early Church had viewed the disease as a punishment for violations of sacred law. St. Ambrose said that the Jews had been eaten away by leprosy of the body and the soul, and the will of St. Ephrem (d. 373) threatened with leprosy anyone who disturbed his remains or doubted the Church.[19] Other Church fathers also saw leprosy as the wages of sin: Jerome claimed it was God's punishment for the original transgression of Adam and Eve, while St. Caesarius of Arles (ca. 470–542) invoked it upon the children of men who violated the chastity the Church required of them during Lent, major festivals, or the pregnancy and menstrual periods of their wives. Gregory of Tours (538–593) told a story about a thief who stole from a church and was stricken with leprosy as a result. Documents from the eleventh and twelfth centuries described leprosy as God's recompense for blasphemous and cruel acts, and Odo of Cheriton (ca. 1180–1247) retold the story of the original sin with a leper in the place of the serpent.

Most of all, leprosy was tied to the sin of lust. This belief, too, had early Christian roots. Lactantius (ca. 250–325, defender of Christianity against Roman attacks) said that those who sinned because of their insatiable desires should be treated as lepers. Rightly or wrongly—physicians still disagree—leprosy was embroiled in a confusion with sexually transmitted diseases, a belief that can be traced back to fifth-century India and was commonplace in twelfth-century European medical writings. Christian authors of the same era, including the profoundly influential St. Bernard of Clairvaux, believed that leprosy afflicted the children of promiscuous parents. By the sixteenth century, some physicians called the disease "satyriasis," believing that it was linked with this state of continuous and painful sexual arousal. The Italian physician Girolamo Fracastoro (1478–1553) even claimed that, because eunuchs rarely suffered from leprosy, some people castrated themselves in a desperate quest for immunity from the dread disease. Medieval laws imposed harsh penalties on lepers who had sex with prostitutes, and a leprosy diagnosis rendered marriages null and void.[20] Some twelfth-century Christian writers, such as Hildegard of Bingen and William of Conches (d. after 1145) even associated leprosy with melancholy, the root cause of lovesickness, saying that the skin disease was caused by an excess of black bile in the blood.

These beliefs ensured that chastity was strictly enforced on lepers. The leper house of Meaux, for example, founded in the late twelfth century, required that a male resident found with a woman at night do humiliating penance by eating bread and water on the ground, "at the master's pleasure." Those who went past simple fraternization and were actually caught *in flagrante delicto* were imprisoned or expelled. In the leper house at Andelys, men who fornicated were expelled for a year and a day from the food and shelter the hospice provided; women who became pregnant were expelled or imprisoned "forever."[21] The house at Lille prohibited not only marriage, but also lust and simple infatuation. Even lepers who had been married were forbidden to have sex—even if their spouses were devoted enough to take up residence in the hospice. Married couples lived and slept apart; their only common activity was the sharing of lunch once a week; all sexual contact was forbidden.

Despite all this, the tie between leprosy and sin was not unequivocal. Jesus himself had dined in the house of Simon the Leper at Bethany (Matthew 26), and his acts of healing lepers were reminders that he wiped away every human sin. Even if leprosy was a punishment, it was one that God could remove—and hence less grave than any mortal sin, as St. Louis (crusader and king of France) pointed out to his skeptical biographer Jean de Joinville (1224?–1317?).[22] Louis, however, was an exceptionally holy man. It is probable that most medieval men and women would have taken their chances with heavenly reckoning to avoid the utter social rejection a diagnosis of leprosy would surely bring on earth.

The Living Dead

The fear and superstition lepers aroused gave them a strange status: they were not members of society, but neither were they altogether out of mind. Both civil and religious law wrestled with this uneasiness and tried to come up with ways of placing these troubled souls into a condition that reflected society's views. Morally, socially, legally, and religiously, lepers were the living dead, whom God had marked out and who could no longer be part of human society, yet who still walked the earth.

From early days, many people believed that lepers were scarcely human—"men already dead except to sin," as St. Gregory Nazianzen put it at St. Basil's funeral in 379. Some Christians tried to redeem their sufferings with promises of a special grace: they argued that lepers were being punished in this life so that they would not have to suffer in the next. Sixth-century Christian councils ordained that the Church should pay for lepers' care; a twelfth-century manuscript spoke of a man who was "marked with leprosy by the will of God." The rules of some leper houses required the residents to fill their days to overflowing with prayers, and perhaps it was in exchange for this spiritual labor that Jacques de Vitry (ca. 1170–1240), in his *History of the West,* promised that God would turn their lives of excrement into precious jewels, and their fetid odor into a sweet fragrance. Leprosy could lead to salvation, as Guy de Chauliac (ca. 1300–1368, the most eminent surgeon of the Middle Ages) averred. But this salvation was reached only through suffering: even Chauliac admitted that the world loathed lepers, and the founders of Finnish leper houses in 1440 and as late as 1619 described the disease as "a divine punishment for sin."[23]

Regardless of whether people—both laymen and ecclesiastics—believed lepers were blessed or cursed, the one thing they were sure of was that they did not want lepers in their towns. Laws expelling them from cities were one attempt to keep their festering sores out of view; building leper houses was another, more charitable, approach. But starker and more chilling were the ceremonies of separation the Church developed in the later Middle Ages to teach lepers to stay out of the lives of ordinary folk and to remind the latter that lepers were truly members of the dead.[24]

First, the leper was wrapped in a shroud; then he or she was carried to a church that had been draped in funereal black, where the priest took a final confession and intoned the solemn liturgy of a requiem mass. The service then moved to the churchyard. Standing in an open grave, the leper was directly addressed by the priest—not in Latin, as usual, but in the vernacular, to avoid any possibility of misunderstanding. Leprosy, explained the priest, was a sign of God's mercy. Rather than waiting until death, the leper was being punished for his or her sins before even departing from this life. Sometimes the priest would scatter a shovelful of earth over the leper's head. The priest then provided the few possessions the invalid would henceforth own. These filled only a short list: a purse, a drinking cup, a food bag, gloves, a cloak, and a wooden clapper, the leper's symbolic new voice, designed to prevent the leper's infecting the air by his or her noisome speech. "See here the tongue the Church has granted you," the priest would explain, "forbidding you to ask for alms except by means of this instrument. And also, the Church forbids you ever to speak to anyone unless you are bidden to speak."

The funeral culminated with the ten commandments the leper had to observe from that point forward—laws that showed how far he or she was banished from the company of others. The priest proclaimed to the entombed leper:

1. I forbid you ever again to enter churches, mills, bakehouses, or markets, or to be found in assemblies of people.
2. Ever to wash your hands, or anything you use, in fountains, rivers, or streams the public employs. I order you that if you want to draw water for your needs, you use your stoup or some other clean vessel for this purpose.
3. I forbid you to leave your house without wearing shoes, your leper's habit, and your clapper, in order that everyone can identify you.
4. To touch anything you want to buy, wherever you are, except with a rod or pole.
5. To enter taverns or other houses for any reason whatsoever; if you want to buy or accept wine from someone, I order that you have it poured into your stoup.
6. To answer questions from anyone you meet on the road unless you are downwind of them, to avoid infecting those you pass.
7. To pass through narrow streets, to avoid contagion by touch.
8. If in traveling you are obliged to urinate, I forbid you to touch the posts and other instruments designated for this purpose, without putting on your gloves first.
9. Ever to touch small children, or to give them anything, or to give anything to any person whatsoever.

10. Ever again to eat or drink in the company of others, except for that of other lepers.

After a few final words of spiritual comfort, the leper was escorted to a special hospice, never to return. His or her will took effect; all property passed to the leper's heirs. Legally widowed, the leper's spouse was free to remarry. The leper was now dead to the world.[25]

Even this was not the limit of lepers' isolation: they were also banished from spiritual life. In the early Middle Ages, there were times when lepers were barred from the sacrament of communion. In some places they were forbidden to enter churches altogether; all they could do was to stare at the mass through a small window designated for their use. And when lepers died, in the Béarn region of France, they were buried silently, at nightfall, away from the bodies of the rest of the congregation—almost as if they had never really been alive.[26]

Civil treatment of lepers echoed that of the Church: secular laws treated the diseased as only partly human. In the twelfth century, some rulers emphasized the holy nature of lepers' not-quite-human status, visiting their hospitals, bathing their sores, and even kissing their hands. As time went on, however, civil society treated lepers more and more harshly. A 1288 law from the Béarn region stated that finding a person guilty of murder required the testimony "of six persons, and if there are none, of thirty *cagots*" (those afflicted with a skin disease considered to be a form of leprosy). A 1329 Scots law ordered that any rotten pork or salmon brought to market was not fit to be sold to the public; instead, it should be given to the leper folk, or else destroyed. At times, lepers' subhuman status meant that they were treated even worse than this: particularly in the fourteenth century, lepers were burnt alive. This exceptional cruelty became possible because tolerance for all minorities (lepers, homosexuals, heretics, Jews) was declining, but another strong motivation was greed. By this time, centuries after their foundation, some leper houses had amassed property and income, and, in order to lay their hands on these revenues, rulers announced that lepers had poisoned municipal wells—and then burned the alleged perpetrators alive. Hospital lands and treasuries then fell like ripe fruit into the grasping hands of the powerful.[27]

SINCE I MUST LEAVE MY HOME

A few personal voices still echo from these sorrowful days. Two poets from the French city of Arras wrote poems of farewell to their friends when they were sent off to live out their days in the leper house of

Grand Val. One was Jean Bodel (d. 1210), a versatile trouvère whose works included lyric poems, an epic about Charlemagne, and a miracle play about St. Nicholas. Bodel concealed his disease from his fellow citizens as long as he could, but eventually his days of liberty came to an end.

The dominant theme of his "Farewell" was sorrow. "I am so melancholy that my heart breaks," he wrote to his friends, thanking them one by one for their kindnesses past: "for nothing makes me so sad as to bid you adieu." Bodel wrote that his life on earth was over; all he could hope was that his sufferings in this world would redeem him in the next. "There is no argument I can make against God," he lamented; all he could do was accept his lot. "Since he has taken my body, I freely give him my soul." He begged God to accept his penance, for to go through this hell and then face another after death would be more than he could bear; the Church's promises of salvation were all the hope he retained.

Sixty years later, the poet Baude Fastoul (d. after 1270) made his way to the same hospice. "I must not turn from my path," he wrote, regretfully, "if God wishes to send me evil to punish my grievous sins. May he guide me to a safe harbor and keep me company on my pilgrimage." Sin and repentance weighed heavily on Fastoul's mind as he prepared his departure: "The disease that keeps me from speaking shows me clearly that I must not live in arrogance or pride. Instead, I must go to a quiet place and pray God with all my heart and faith, for unless I repent I have no worth." In the anxiety of Fastoul's "Farewell," there are glimmers of sorrowful hope. He prayed that his rotting body would smell sweetly before God, and he prayed, in language that would be echoed centuries later by English ministers writing about the plague, that even as his body weakened, his heart was in the care of a physician who could heal it when the rest was lost. As he gave up his place in this world, Baude Fastoul hoped he would find a happier one in the world to come.

A contemporary of Fastoul's, the poet and playwright Adam de la Halle (d. 1286 or 1287) borrowed the genre of the lepers' farewell when he left Arras to head into exile. The haunting images he evoked reminded readers of all the earthly beauty lepers had to leave behind as they headed off to their solitary shelter. "Since I must leave my home," wrote Adam,

> Farewell, Hauiel, farewell Robert Nasart. Farewell, Gilles le Père, farewell Jean Joie. You never missed a joust; you spent your gold on lances, tipped with beautiful banners of silk and cloth of gold. Alas, the good city where I used to see men joust for honor on the playing field is silent now.

And yet—it seems as if I still can see the fiery air aflame with your
pennant-tipped lances and your games.[28]

The thirteenth and fourteenth centuries were cruel times for many—
even those without leprosy. People were hanged for stealing; outlaws
could be beaten or killed as freely as dogs; courts sentenced criminals
to be dragged to death, beheaded, and even buried alive. At times the
blind were treated as a spectacle, paraded through the streets or forced
into combat with one another.[29] It was not good to depend on the
tender mercies of the public in the late Middle Ages.

Still, no matter how others suffered, it seems likely that lepers
suffered more. Their bodies decayed, their faces twisted, their hoarse
and honking voices silenced, they wandered from place to place, wanted
nowhere and often tolerated less than the garbage and excrement at the
side of the road. Cut off from their families (unless these had enough
money to keep them in isolation at home), they lost not only their
earthly property, their livelihood, their spouses, but also their access to
communities of the spirit.

Though it has largely died out in temperate countries—driven out
by tuberculosis, argue some medical authorities—leprosy continues to
afflict two million people worldwide. Most are in Asia, Africa, and
Central and South America, though leper communities also remain in
Hawai'i; the last one in the continental United States, in Carville, Loui-
siana, is closing now. Physicians agree that the disease is contagious,
though slowly, through prolonged, intimate contact; children of infected parents are particularly susceptible. Antibiotics can treat the disease, and, recently, the long-banned drug thalidomide has shown some
effectiveness. Separating the infected from the rest of the population
can be effective in preventing the spread of the disease. Thus medieval
leper houses may have served some purpose, though most lepers probably were isolated too late to protect their families.

Leper houses must have been some small comfort, as long as the rul-
ing classes did not cast a greedy eye on their property and burn their
inhabitants to death. Perhaps the promises of the priests came true for
some: that by suffering a true purgatory on earth, the afflicted would
find their way to purity more quickly than others. For others, though,
these hints of salvation to come can hardly have made up for the loneli-
ness of living as if they were dead. The fear of lepers, and the memories
of what they suffered, have haunted the West for centuries, and provided an easy—if unfortunate—model to follow when other diseases
came along.

The most striking testimony to this fact was the way lepers haunted

European memory long after the disease had died out in most parts of Europe. To be a leper was the most loathsome and fearful torment that could be imagined, and to be treated like one the greatest punishment society could inflict. The tie between leprosy and sexual sin remained strong in the popular imagination: the immensely popular sixteenth-century Catholic preacher Michel Menot (ca. 1440–1518) would describe syphilitics as "leprous and stinking"; so would John Calvin. This was no poetic metaphor: in the sixteenth and seventeenth centuries, in Tours, Ulm, Alcmaer, Vienna, and Glasgow, medieval leper hospitals were thrust back into use to contain the lepers' wretched heirs—those who suffered from the new scourge of syphilis.[30] Long after the people they were meant to house had died, these decrepit and ominous buildings kept their memory alive as a warning of the penalty society could impose on those it most loathed and feared.

CHAPTER THREE

The Just Rewards of Unbridled Lust: Syphilis in

Early Modern Europe

Shortly after Christopher Columbus and his sailors returned from their voyage to the New World, a horrifying new disease began to make its way around the Old. The "pox," as it was often called, erupted with dramatic severity. According to Ulrich von Hutten (1488–1523), a German knight, revolutionary, and author who wrote a popular book about his own trials with syphilis and the treatments he underwent, the first European sufferers were covered with acorn-sized boils that emitted a foul, dark green pus. This secretion was so vile, von Hutten affirmed, that even the burning pains of the boils troubled the sick less than their horror at the sight of their own bodies. Yet this was only the beginning. People's flesh and skin filled with water; their bladders developed sores; their stomachs were eaten away. Girolamo Fracastoro, a professor at the University of Padua, described the onward march of symptoms: syphilis pustules developed into ulcers that dissolved skin, muscle, bone, palate, and tonsils—even lips, noses, eyes, and genital organs. Rubbery tumors, filled with a white, sticky mucus, grew to the size of rolls of bread. Violent pains tormented the afflicted, who were exhausted but could not sleep, and suffered starvation without feeling hunger. Many of them died.

The public was appalled by this scourge. Physicians too, von Hutten reported, were so revolted that they would not even touch their patients. As in the earlier Middle Ages, divines quickly announced that the extraordinary sins of the age were responsible for the new plague; others blamed the stars, miasmas, and various other causes. Barrels of medical ink were spilled on the question of where the disease had come from. Treatments, preventions, and cures were sought. The idea of infection began to be taken far more seriously than it ever had before. Hospitals transformed themselves in response to the new plague—sometimes for the better, but often for the worse, as when, in fear, they cast their ulcerated patients out into the streets. Most of all, people continued to follow their old ways: in the face of this new threat, they castigated and persecuted the sick. As infection spread, so did fear; and where fear went, blame followed close behind.

Perhaps more than any other disease before or since, syphilis in early modern Europe provoked the kind of widespread moral panic that AIDS revived when it struck America in the 1980s. Syphilitics were condemned from pulpits and from chairs in university medical schools. John Calvin (1509–1564) announced that "God has raised up new diseases against debauchery";[1] medical authorities willingly agreed. The greatest English surgeon of the sixteenth century, William Clowes (1540–1604), who counted Queen Elizabeth among his patients, announced to his colleagues and patients that syphilis was "loathsome and odious, yea troublesome and dangerous, a notable testimony of the just wrath of God." A century later, a French physician, M. Flamand, summed up this point of view concisely by announcing that venereal diseases were "the just rewards of unbridled lust." Disease commonly invited theological speculation, but in the case of syphilis people felt that little speculation was necessary. Just as fornication opened the door to the pox, so the pox opened the door to chastisement and blame.

Motivated by these fears, panicky towns and hospitals barred their gates against syphilitics. Within two years of the first reported cases, cities from Geneva to Aberdeen evicted the pox-ridden. Often, city fathers blamed prostitutes for the disease, and some threatened to brand their cheeks with hot iron if they did not desist from their vices.[2] Sexual morality was becoming stricter, and prostitutes were usually condemned far more savagely than the men who used their services.

What was more extraordinary, however, was that hospitals refused to admit syphilis patients. Hospitals in early modern Europe were charitable institutions, designed to provide care and shelter to the sick poor. The most famous of them, the Paris Hôtel-Dieu prided itself, with one single exception, on the breadth of its generosity. This hospital boasted that it "receives, feeds, and tends all poor sufferers, wherever they come from and whatever ailment they may have, even plague victims—though not if they have the pox."[3] The Hôtel-Dieu expelled its syphilitic patients in 1496, and, after relenting briefly, expelled them again in 1508. Two years after that, another Parisian hospital shunted its pox victims off to the stables, to sleep with the animals. Many cities threw the poxy poor into the leper houses that for years and years had housed only ghostly memories; Toulouse kept its infected prostitutes in a ward that was little more than a high-security prison. Two infamous hospitals in Paris, Bicêtre and the Salpêtrière, had patients "piled upon one another," in the words of historian Michel Mollat, "like a cargo of Negroes in an African slave ship." And another, the Petites Maisons, which warehoused syphilitics and the mentally ill from the 1550s until the 1800s, became known as the "pox-victims' Bastille."[4]

Fear of contact was one reason for this behavior. Even more than this, however, the sick—like lepers—were often reviled because people believed that they had brought their torments upon themselves. Some pundits, early on, announced that blasphemy was the vice that had called down this new torment from heaven, but most often syphilis was attributed to the sin of lust. This was certainly a logical assumption: soldiers and prostitutes, traditionally associated with sexual license and moral disorder, were among the first victims, and the connection became even closer when people noticed that the disease's first sores often turned up on the genital organs. The loathsome symptoms were taken as signs that the sick housed debauched and sinful souls. This reasoning stood behind many of the cruelties that individuals, doctors, hospitals, priests, ministers, and even entire towns and cities inflicted on people with the pox, as the stories in this chapter will show.

THE SOURCE OF THIS DISTEMPER

Horror was the first emotion the pox provoked among the general public, but what the medical community first felt was confusion. Was this an old disease, and, if so, which one? If it was new, what did that say about the state of medical knowledge? And in any case, how could physicians make sense of it?

Medical research in the twentieth century mostly takes place in the lab; in the Renaissance, though, researchers went first and foremost to the library to see what the ancients had said. The problem, however, was that it was not clear that in this case the ancients had anything useful to offer. Nothing the Greek and Arabic authorities had described seemed very similar to the cases turning up in increasing numbers on the physicians' rounds and in the streets, and so it was hard to affirm that the old remedies would do any good.

If the pox was a new disease, how had it arisen? Some cast the blame on supernatural powers—the planets, the stars, God, or even witches. Galenists claimed that the pox came from corrupted air, or even, like lovesickness, from an excess of black bile.[5] Some said the disease was God's punishment for sin; others attributed it to the recent and risky voyages to the New World.

The theories that tied the disease to the Americas were the most innovative, since they focused on the new idea that diseases could travel from one person to another. (They may also have been the most accurate: many scientists today believe that the New World was the source of the syphilis bacterium, or of a new strain or cofactor that triggered the epidemic of the 1490s.) In a quirky 1672 screed entitled *Great Venus Unmasked,* the English writer Gideon Harvey looked backward to argue that it was Columbus's Neapolitan sailors who had acquired this "new pretty toy." With it, he reasoned, they had infected the prostitutes of their native city, which was under siege by the French in 1494–1495: when provisions in Naples ran out, wrote Harvey, the whores crept over to the besiegers' camp, and offered their services to the French soldiers. If the Neapolitan prostitutes were hungry for food, Harvey explained, the French soldiers were "almost starved for want of women's flesh, which they found so well seasoned, and daubed with mustard, that in a few weeks it took 'em all by the nose."

Other exotic theories abounded. One Leonardo Fioravanti (1518–1588) claimed that the French soldiers became sick because they had devoured the rotten carcasses of their dead enemies. Some said the malady had been bred when a French leper had sex with a Neapolitan whore. Others said soldiers became sick from drinking Greek wine adulterated with lepers' blood; still others blamed the "entailed manginess" of the French, who—as Harvey reminded his English readers— "are slovens in their linen." One anonymous author even suggested that syphilis was spontaneously generated by promiscuous sex.[6]

This wild proliferation of theories showed that nobody really knew where the pox had come from; it also showed that people were deeply troubled by it, and thought that something had gone gravely amiss in the world to provoke such a strange and awful evil. Their confusion and anxiety were also revealed by the names that people gave the new arrival. The name most commonly used today, syphilis, came from an Italian poem, written in 1530, which traced the disease to a punishment inflicted by Jupiter on a fictional character named Syphilus, an impious shepherd. More commonly, however, the pox was called after whichever country people wanted to blame for the disease. To the French, it was the *mal de Naples,* the sickness from Naples; to many others, it was the *morbus gallicus,* the French disease. But also accused were the Americans, the Mexicans, the Spanish, the Germans, the Poles, and the Portuguese. Everyone, observed the astute author of *A New Method of Curing the French-Pox* (1690), "to excuse himself, is forward to ascribe to his neighbors the source and original of this distemper."

Regardless of its geographic origin, people quickly began to notice that the pox traveled from one person to another. They sometimes blamed transmission on common and morally innocuous practices—drinking from a common cup, kissing friends in church, following a syphilitic comrade on the latrine.[7] But from 1495 on, the route of transmission people talked about most was sex. Von Hutten noticed that men in their sexually active years were much more susceptible to the French disease than boys or the elderly; soldiers and prostitutes remained highly suspect. As early as 1504, infection became grounds for breaking off engagements, and even saying that someone was infected was enough to provoke a lawsuit.[8] Syphilis was well on its way to becoming a "venereal" disease, and a public mark of shame.

A Moral Revolution

It seems likely that these developments were related to a dramatic change of moral climate that was sweeping over Europe. Though it is impossible to know all the details of this picture, particularly five hundred years after the fact, an educated guess would suggest that this major new public health problem contributed to people's increasingly negative attitudes toward sex, a shift in views that revolutionized people's lives. For heterosexual men, at least, the 1400s had been an era of comparatively free sexuality. In part, this was because people married late: men often waited to wive until their fathers had died and left property and businesses to them. As a result, many men remained unmarried long after they reached sexual maturity, and a male-dominated social structure left these single men free to find ways to satisfy their urges.

Historical records show that young men had a number of common sexual outlets. One was masturbation, which young men (though not young women) could practice without attracting much condemnation. Another was rape. Young men—groups of adolescents, especially—frequently assaulted poor girls who had no male protection, and the perpetrators generally suffered far less than their victims for the consequences of their actions. For example, in the little city of Dijon, which in the fifteenth century contained fewer than three thousand households, at least twenty rapes were reported every year.[9] Who knows how many more actually occurred? More commonly still, men used prostitutes, whether these were elegant courtesans, whores they met in the brothels or—even further down the social ladder—poor women who made a seedy living servicing male customers at the baths. Men scarcely needed to be married to have sex.

Women were not necessarily sexually monogamous either, though when they were promiscuous it was often less out of choice than from obligation, whether through rape or the force of circumstances. In theory, girls remained virgins until they were married, passing directly from their fathers' control to their husbands'; in practice, however, many did not manage to remain on this straight and narrow path. Rape was one common ambush, especially for poor girls, and this often led them even further afield, to prostitution. The same was true of girls who had lost their place in society by being orphaned, wives who fled husbands who abused them, and women who were discharged, penniless, from public hospitals. The oldest profession extended its lucrative embrace to the homeless, the victimized, and the poor.

Prostitution was not a very respectable way for women to earn a living in the fifteenth century, but it was not exceptionally shameful, and it paid well. In half an hour, a prostitute could make as much money as a woman laboring in a vineyard could earn in half a day.[10] The financial rewards were so tempting, in fact, that in lean times even married women sometimes joined this labor force.

In addition, prostitution was tolerated, and often even actively promoted, by town and church leaders, who felt that society would collapse if unmarried men did not have this squalid but essential outlet for their sexual desires. This view had a prestigious heritage, having been articulated by none other than St. Augustine. Before his conversion to Christianity, Augustine had accumulated substantial experience in the pleasures of the flesh, as witnessed by his famous prayer, "Lord, give me chastity and continence—but not just yet." Even in his maturer years, the saint felt that men's nature was such that whores were an unfortunate social necessity. "What is more sordid, more worthless, more full of shame and disgrace than prostitutes, pimps, and other plagues of this kind?" Augustine rhetorically inquired, disapproval dripping from his episcopal pen. "If, however," he went on to warn, "you remove prostitutes from human society, you will overturn everything with lust."[11] Prostitution, Augustine argued, was like a city sewer system—disgusting, but essential to maintaining cleanliness and order in every other area.

Late medieval town leaders even argued that prostitution was a public good—perhaps because it was a way to appease the sexual urges of the working men the upper classes had driven out of the marriage market. Cities owned and operated brothels. Bishops and abbots owned bathhouses, and supported themselves on their profits; the fact that these establishments made getting dirty as much fun as getting clean was not considered a problem. Many clergymen, in fact, were among the baths' and brothels' clientele: at certain times and in certain places, in fact, one customer in five was a cleric.[12]

In the early 1500s, however, chillier moral winds began to blow. The public, which in the past had tolerated brothels as a fact of life, began to consider them shameful. Prostitutes were denounced and arrested; the Bishop of Winchester's London bordellos were shut down. French cities closed their brothels; Geneva expelled its whores. The freeze affected more than just prostitutes; increasingly, women in general were blamed as a corrupting influence on men.[13] And in 1539, only five years after its creation, Michelangelo's *Last Judgment* was declared obscene; the offending parts were painted over. Old-fashioned sexual license was as out of place in this new era as painted and gilded statues of the Virgin Mary and the saints would have been in an austerely undecorated Protestant church.

Part of this change was the result of religious developments. Protestants made much of the sins of the flesh: lust so afflicted humankind, preached Martin Luther (1483–1546), that God had been obliged to create matrimony as "a hospital for incurables." Calvin saw sexual vices everywhere: the young, he preached, were tormented by "boiling affections," while fornicators were pigs who soiled the very blood of Christ by mixing it with "the stinking mire." Even in the holy city of Geneva—even in his own church council—Calvin believed he was surrounded by "fornicators, wife-beaters, idolaters, and heretics."[14]

Did syphilis contribute to these changes? Obviously, not all can be attributed to the new disease: the rise of Protestantism was a far larger and more influential matter than any bacterium. But a new, virulent, sexually transmitted infection can only have reinforced people's increasing fears and anxieties about sex.[15]

Neither preachers nor physicians had the slightest hesitation about announcing that syphilis—and syphilitics—were wicked. Both Catholics and Protestants endorsed this view and proclaimed it from their pulpits. One of the most popular Catholic preachers of the day, a Franciscan monk named Michel Menot, focused on the "Naples pox" in a sermon delivered during the penitential Lenten season of 1508. The sins of the flesh, proclaimed Brother Michel, made the body leprous, stinking, and infirm; the pox simply worked God's will. "Lust shortens the days of mankind," he concluded, Q.E.D. The Catholic queen of Navarre, Marguérite d'Angoulême (1492–1549), agreed. Fornication led to infection, she wrote in her poetic confession, *The Mirror of a Sinful Soul* (1531), a book Elizabeth I of England (1533–1603) found so moving and persuasive that she translated it into English herself.

Protestants also enthusiastically linked sickness with immorality: Calvin warned Geneva that the new and strange diseases showed clearly that "God is more angry than ever" with the sins of humankind.[16] A century later, in England, Edward Lawrence (1623–1695) phrased the same sentiment in even more inflammatory language. Through the filthy sin of whoredom, he fulminated, "men and women sacrifice their health, estates, names, bodies, and souls to their stinking lusts, carrying a filthy and guilty soul in a rotten body whilst they live, and shutting themselves out of heaven and into hell when they die." The torments of the body merely showed the public the inner degradation of the soul.

THE MORALITY OF MEDICINE

Some physicians took a more tolerant stance than these vitriolic preachers. Others, however, were even more censorious than the men of the cloth, and warned that pox victims were so sinful that they did not even deserve medical treatment. Syphilis revived the old questions that lovesickness had raised centuries before: should the doctor do what was best for his patients' bodies, or should he attend to their souls? If they tried to care for both, would there be conflicts? And when the patient's life was at stake, which side would win?

Like attitudes throughout society, doctors' views on syphilis grew more severe as time went on. Few physicians ever felt that syphilis was a morally neutral issue, but some of the earliest writers were at least willing to separate their spiritual concerns from their medical practice. For example, Johannes Widman (professor at the University of Tübingen, ca. 1460–ca. 1500), wrote around 1500 that "a doctor, as a doctor, does not cure much" by arguing about whether a disease is caused by human sin or by the wheeling of the constellations in the heavens. If doctors simply removed the bodily causes of disease, he asserted, their patients would recover far more quickly than if the doctor tried to redeem his patient's virtue first.

Widman's willingness to cure the pox was seconded by Gaspare Torrella (1440–1524), a Spanish physician who was also a bishop. Ever a self-promoter, Torrella reassured his readers that, "with the help of all-powerful God and his mother, the most glorious Virgin Mary, the pox can be cured if the doctor is clever and follows all the instructions I provide." Torrella's close ties with the Borgia family—not a notoriously clean-living bunch—may have taught him tolerance, or at least expedience: within a single two-month period, the doctor-bishop treated for syphilis not only the cardinal of Valencia, who happened to be Pope Alexander VI's illegitimate son, but also seventeen other Borgias and members of the papal court. Presumably, Torrella understood that it did not pay to preach at the pope's family.[17] A physician from Geneva, Jacobus Catenus de Lacumarino, also argued (around 1504) that he had an obligation to treat syphilitics, regardless of how they had become infected. For these men, religious morality did not necessarily determine how they carried out their professional responsibilities.

Other doctors, however, feared the hand of God they saw in this disease. The famous anatomist Gabriel Fallopius (1523–1562), who had succeeded to Vesalius's chair at the University of Padua, announced that God had sent the "French scab" expressly to teach people to beware his wrath and abandon venereal lust. Juan Almenar (another of Pope Alexander VI's doctors, fl. ca. 1500), believed that vices and diseases came in pairs, like the animals on Noah's ark. Thus pride was matched with fever, sloth with gout, and lust with leprosy and its modern reincarnation, the pox. These views—a throwback to ancient ideas of disease that are still echoed by the self-help preacher-healers of today—made offering a cure a moral dilemma: what if doing so endangered the patient's soul—not to mention that of the doctor, who fostered sin by curing the afflictions it caused?

Sin also haunted those Englishmen who wrote on syphilis. English doctors feared that if they provided medical care to those "wicked and sinful creatures" who brought this disease down upon themselves, the abetting physicians would be standing directly in the way of God's will. William Clowes, for example, had no interest in encouraging "rogues and idle persons, men and women," to wallow in the muck and continue to live the beastly lives that had made them sick. He published his remedies, he explained, only for the honest and the good. His contemporary William Bullein (d. 1576), an English physician and botanist, read his lesson from the same text. No one who had gotten sick with the "filthy, rotten burning of harlots," Bullein argued, had any right to seek a cure: such people should not even expect to find one in his book. He provided his remedies only for the blameless, the ignorant, and the unfortunate—those who had contracted the pox through no fault of their own.

The rest would have to suffer. These views were fully backed by the greatest scientific laureates of the day, such as the French surgeon Ambroise Paré (ca. 1510–1590) and the Flemish chemist and physicist Jan Baptista van Helmont (1577–1644). They too were convinced that syphilis was God's way of punishing the deadly and all-too-human affliction of lust.

INNOCENT VICTIMS

The fact that babies and faithful wives could contract syphilis made it impossible to condemn every single person who came down with the disease. But babies had little in common, surely, with prostitutes and adulterers, so medical authorities divided syphilitics into two groups, and treated them accordingly: the "guilty," who had earned the pox by their sinful behavior, and the "innocent," who had done nothing to deserve it. Along with drugs, these physicians also dispensed moral advice that would provide a model for social views of venereal disease in the centuries to come.

Medical writers' remarks on syphilis were a real window into their views of human nature. Some tolerance, for example, was shown by the English doctor "L.S.," author of a book called *Prophylaktikon* (1673). He reminded his fellow doctors to show patience to men who had been led by passion to commit foolish acts. The debauched husband and his lusts were detestable, of course; still, L.S. could find it in his heart to hate such a man's sin while yet loving the sinner. But the prostitutes who led these men to their destruction—theirs was a different story: the milk of this physician's kindness curdled in his breast when he thought of these pocky and infectious whores. If he had his wish, Dr. S. wrote, prostitutes would do themselves a favor and die of the pox, or do a courtesy to humankind and hang themselves. And if fortune was not so cooperative—well, Dr. S. had a remedy of his own to suggest: why not transport all the infected prostitutes away from England to the royal plantations in the New World? There they could engage in productive work, while the balmy climate improved their health. There was an added bonus, as well: the example of these sinful whores, ripped from the breast of Mother England, would terrorize lustful women and, perhaps, "fright them into better manners." Men could be cured, but wicked women must be sent far away.

The good and the wicked received their own due justice from a French medical moralist, too. In her *Collection of Easy and Domestic Remedies* (1678), Marie de Maupeou Fouquet (1590–1681) made it clear that venereal diseases were different from others. In most of her book's entries, Mme. Fouquet would simply list a disease's symptoms, and then offer a few home remedies that would cure the ill without straining a middle-class pocketbook. Venereal diseases, however, provoked a fierce and furious sermon. These ills, she explained, were not simply a health problem, but rather the natural and just consequences of the most fatal of sins, the sin that "sent more souls tumbling headlong into hell than all others combined." The proper way to treat the venereally afflicted, she declared, was not to comfort them with mild remedies, but instead to increase their torments by meting out the rigorous penances they deserved. Mme. Fouquet's flinty sense of justice, however, was melted by the warmth of divine mercy (on which, perhaps, she had learned to rely as she suffered through the long, public, and scandalous embezzlement trial of her son, Louis XIV's discredited minister of finances). Charity toward the innocent victims of syphilis led Mme. Fouquet to offer remedies for the pox, even though the guilty would unfairly benefit as a result of her kindness.

WORSE THAN THE DISEASE

Treatments for the pox were often more excruciating than the disease's symptoms. According to their place in society, early modern Europeans received varying types of medical care, but all were problematic. The rich were seen by physicians, whose treatments ranged from the useless to the deadly; the middle classes could consult self-help books, or hire barber-surgeons to torture them with knives, drills, and white-hot cautery irons. The poor had to deal with charity hospitals. If admitted to these institutions, they were housed and fed, but they also shared beds and germs with all the other diseased patients in their wards, and often received little medical help; if they were refused admission, they suffered and died in the streets. It was hard to say which was worse—to languish untreated, as syphilis ate its way through one's organs, or to be tortured by poisonous and savage remedies administered by physicians and surgeons who often believed that their job was to punish their patients for their sins. To have syphilis in early modern Europe was a torment and a tragedy for rich and poor alike.

Doctors did not use harsh remedies at first, perhaps because the disease had not yet earned real opprobrium, or perhaps because these early cures derived from the Galenic model, which, whatever its limitations, at least employed fairly gentle methods. Physicians who viewed the disease as a humoral imbalance recommended baths, chicken broth, bloodletting, syrups, the milk of a woman who had given birth to a daughter, and even that old standby used for curing lovesickness, sexual intercourse.[18] (This last piece of medical foolishness, fortunately, did not garner many endorsements.) Others warned of the dangers of promiscuous sex, particularly with prostitutes; some even proposed safer sex techniques for preventing the pox, such as washing the genitals, before or after intercourse, in hot vinegar or white wine. It probably took physicians a while to realize that these mild remedies, while doing no harm, did little good, either. Syphilis was new, after all, and nobody knew at first that the disease passed through primary, secondary, and tertiary stages, each with distinct symptoms and with quiescent periods in between. Eventually, though, physicians did realize that they were doing their patients no particular service with remedies of this sort.[19]

Gradually doctors came to understand that, once acquired, syphilis tended to persist, and gradually its severe symptoms and venereal taint attracted much more aggressive medical treatment. Some doctors, for example, injected drugs directly into male patients' infected urethras. A character in the writings of the Dutch humanist scholar Desiderius Erasmus (1469–1536) spoke in favor of binding female syphilitics in chastity belts, and of deporting, castrating, and even burning poxridden men alive. Surgeons treated racking syphilis headaches by trepanation, the ancient practice of boring holes into the skull. Oozing ulcers in skin and bone were cauterized with fearsome, white-hot irons.[20] Mild remedies quickly gave way to these treatments, which at least showed that doctors were doing something their patients could *feel.*

THESE BITTER PAINS AND EVILS

Bleeding, bathing, cautery, and herbs were used now and then, but, most often, physicians fought syphilis with two important drugs: mercury, and the wood of the Central American guaiac, or *lignum vitae,* tree. Ulrich von Hutten was well acquainted with these, having suffered through the appalling mercury vapor treatment eleven times in nine years. As he explained the process in his book, patients were shut in a "stew," a small steam room, for twenty or thirty days at a time. Seated or lying down, they were spread from head to foot with a mercury-based ointment, swathed in blankets, and left until the sweat poured down; often they fainted from the heat. Disgusting secretions issued from their mouths and noses; sores filled their throats and tongues,

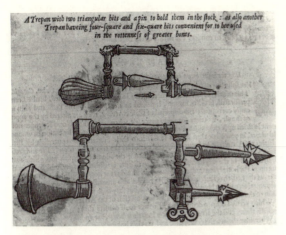

A Trepan with two triangular bits and a pin to hold them in the stock : as also another Trepan haveing four-square and six-quare bits convenient for to bee used in the rottennes of greater bones.

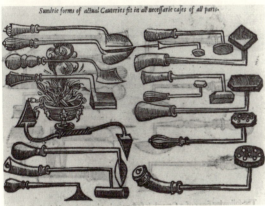

Sundrie forms of actual Cauteries fit in all necessarie cases of all parts.

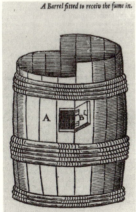

A Barrel fitted to receiv the fume in.

Trepan (tool for drilling holes in the skull); cautery irons; a barrel for inhaling mercury fumes. From *The Works of That Famous Chirurgion Ambrose Parey,* trans. Thomas Johnson (London, 1649). Courtesy of Archives & Special Collections, Columbia University Health Sciences Division.

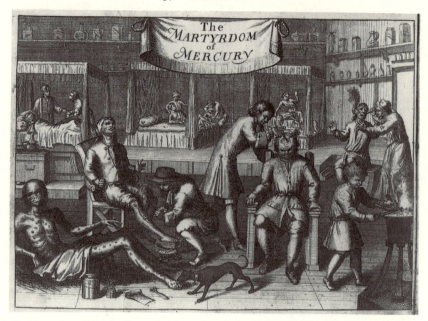

The Martyrdom of Mercury. Treatments for syphilis. J. Sintelaer, *The Scourge of Venus and Mercury, From a Treatise on the Venereal Disease* (London: G. Harris, 1709). Courtesy of the Wellcome Trust Medical Photographic Library, London.

their cheeks and lips, and the rooves of their mouths. Their jaws swelled; often their teeth fell out. Everything stank.

Many patients, von Hutten observed, decided they would rather die than undergo this torture. Others went through it, and died as a result. Von Hutten knew of one anointer, for example, who killed three men in a single day by overheating the stew. His patients suffered silently, believing that, the hotter the room, the sooner they would be cured; but though their patience lasted, their hearts gave way under the strain. Others strangled when their throats swelled so much from mercury poisoning that they could not breathe. And others still died of kidney failure when their urination was blocked too long. "Very few there were," von Hutten lamented, "that got their health, if they passed through these jeopardies, these bitter pains and evils."

Stranger methods for applying mercury were dreamed up, too. It could be taken internally, for example: one eighteenth-century recipe called for mixing the liquid metal with hot chocolate, though the author cautioned against this exotic beverage because he felt that the *chocolate* was too dangerous for those afflicted with the French disease. One entrepreneurial medic marketed underpants coated inside with a mercury ointment.[21] All these remedies were based on the theory that, once inside the body, quicksilver atoms spread through it, eliminating the "pocky miasmas" through sweat and the copious salivation that the heavy metal provoked.

These doctors were not wrong about the virtues of mercury, which Arab physicians had used for centuries to treat diseases of the skin: mercury kills the syphilis bacterium *in vitro,* and it may also help the body's immune system to attack the microorganism. The problem, however, is that mercury is a deadly poison, particularly in vapor form or when combined with other substances. (Mercuric chloride, for example, commonly prescribed as "corrosive sublimate" in early modern medical handbooks, is fatal in doses as small as a single gram.) Von Hutten correctly noted such symptoms of mercury poisoning as excessive salivation, loosening of the teeth, pain and numbness in the extremities, uremia, and renal damage; other toxic effects include vomiting, dizziness, convulsions, tremors, liver damage, anorexia, severe diarrhea, and mental deterioration.[22] This remedy may have helped cure skin problems, but it also hastened syphilitics to their death.

Doctors warned of these dangers as early as the 1490s. Bishop Torrella, for example, noted that mercury had killed numerous syphilis patients he knew of, including a cardinal and two members of the Borgia family. Others cautioned against excessive and internal use. But despite the suffering it caused—if not because of it—many physicians enthusiastically endorsed mercury in all its forms, and patients continued to seek out and undergo these treatments, at the cost of their financial resources, their remaining health, and, often, their lives.[23]

In 1517 a much-heralded new treatment for syphilis arrived in Europe, championed by many as less deadly and more effective than mercury. Von Hutten was one of these champions: his book about his experiences of syphilis was an enthusiastic testimonial for the new wonder drug, which he also endorsed as a remedy for gallstones, palsy, leprosy, dropsy, epilepsy, and gout. If we ought to give thanks upward to God for all the good and evil in this life, urged von Hutten, how much more grateful we must be for the mercy God had shown in granting us this happy remedy!

Many echoed these sentiments, reasoning that a New World medicine must be sovereign against what was perceived as a New World disease. Guaiac wood and bark were imported into Europe at staggering prices by a monopoly controlled by the House of Fugger, a mining and banking family who were the Rockefellers of their day. The syphilitic rich imbibed guaiac cocktails as often as they could, and the city of Strasbourg even provided these decoctions free of charge to all of its citizens who were afflicted with the pox.

There were, however, two drawbacks to guaiac. One was that, in actuality, it had no effect against syphilis; about all it did was to induce sweating. (The cynical and eccentric physician-alchemist Paracelsus [1493–1541] suggested—cynically but perhaps accurately—that the only people who benefited from the use of guaiac were the Fuggers.) The other problem was that the regimen under which this new drug was administered was almost as harsh as the awful mercury cure. Patients were once again installed in small heated rooms; they were placed on a rigid diet, or even kept from eating anything at all. Purged with powerful laxatives, they drank large doses of the decoction and sweated profusely for thirty or forty days in a row. Von Hutten cautioned that wine and women were to be strictly avoided during this time, lest such moral impurities anger the generous God who had provided this cure. The punitive nature of the remedy was shown even more strongly by a strange book written in 1527 by Dr. Jacques de Béthencourt, *The New Lent of Penance.* This treatise featured an argument between guaiac and mercury over which one of them cured syphilis more effectively—and which had the dubious merit of making patients suffer more in the process. Syphilitic bodies had to be purified of the disease, but they also needed to be taught a lesson; the harsher that lesson, medics obviously believed, the better.[24]

STRICT CHARITY

For better or worse, not everyone had access to these treatments. The drugs were dreadfully expensive, and a doctor's visit could cost even more. In seventeenth-century England, for example, a single appearance by a physician might cost twenty times the daily income of a poor family of seven. Who could give up enough bread to pay such fees? The middle classes relied on healers with less formal training—surgeons, midwives, herbalists, and so on—and on the increasingly popular medium of the medical self-help book, which retailed to a popular audience the drugs and the judgmental attitudes that physicians could deliver personally to the wealthy. But it was the poor who received the largest dose of spiritual direction when they went to seek health care. This was true, most of all, in French hospitals, of which the most important by far was the Paris Hôtel-Dieu, the hospital that barred syphilis patients from its gates in 1496. On the face of things, it was shocking that the Hôtel-Dieu refused to admit these men and women, since the institution was far more tolerant than almost any other of its time. In subtler ways, however, the Hôtel-Dieu's treatment of syphilis patients simply revealed the pervasive and underlying flaws and weaknesses of the era's medical care for the poor.

Did this religious orientation affect the treatment of patients suffering from the physical and moral scourge of syphilis? It seems likely. Why else would hospitals admit plague victims, swollen, vomiting, and quick to die, yet turn away from those afflicted with the pox? It was not a question of the patients' adherence to the one true faith: the Hôtel-Dieu took in not only Christians, but even Moslems and Jews, and kept an assortment of clergymen on staff to tend to their spiritual needs. The pox, however, was evidence of a kind of sin the hospital feared even more than heresy or death.

True, there were complicating factors. Hospitals generally tried to avoid taking in patients with chronic or incurable diseases. Then as now, hospitals preferred those who would recover quickly, and who would not be a long-term drain on their resources. Moreover, syphilis arrived at a particularly inconvenient time. French hospitals had been badly hurt by the long financial depression caused by the Hundred Years' War (1337–1453), and, starting in the 1490s, the Paris Hôtel-Dieu was racked by accounting scandals and ferocious staff disputes; one unpopular new purser was greeted, on his first day of work, with insults, daggers, and an axe. The ecclesiastical mismanagement and corruption were so appalling, in fact, that over the first decades of the 1500s, public officials took these hospitals over and barred churchmen from holding any administrative posts.[25] The last thing these chaotic institutions needed was a new onslaught of patients afflicted with a virulent, contagious, and disgusting venereal disease.

Most of all, however, syphilis patients were turned away because their disease was a moral problem so severe that it barred even charity itself. Part of this rejection was caused by revulsion; part was caused by the fact that charity was becoming a much more selective enterprise than it had been. Starting in the 1500s, those who gave imposed increasingly high moral standards on those who received, and poor syphilitics were obvious targets for the judgmental upper classes. In the Middle Ages, giving away money had been seen as a virtuous end in itself, and monasteries and the rich willingly distributed largesse. But this system, though based in generosity, was often ineffectual: it had no mechanisms to ensure that money went where it was most needed. As the Middle Ages gave way to the Renaissance, and close-knit feudal society yielded to capitalist economies, rich and poor led increasingly separate lives. Inflation increased, and so did begging—and crime. Charity was viewed, more and more, as a way to control social problems linked with the poor.[26]

The Protestant Reformation played its part in these changing attitudes. Luther constantly reminded those with means that they had to care for those without, but he also stressed the moral responsibilities of the poor. Writing on welfare reform in 1520, he reminded the public of St. Paul's dictum "Whoever will not work shall not eat." Cities had to care for the unfortunate, said Luther, but they also had the right to determine who was truly deserving and who was not. The poor who passed muster were given food and services; the rest (foreigners, malingerers, the idle) were driven away, ridiculed, punished, or even locked up. Women who were considered to be "in danger of becoming lost" were carted off to institutions for "correction," sometimes at the instigation of their husbands. Seventeenth-century English laws ordered that vagabonds be whipped and paraded through town with the letter "V" fastened to their breast, a model for Hawthorne's adulterous Hester Prynne and her scarlet "A." A 1635 English legal handbook distinguished those who were "poor by impotency and defect" (the blind, the lame, the aged, the diseased) and the "poor by casualty" (the victims of accidents, etc.) from "the thriftless poor"—the slothful, the dissolute, vagabonds, and drunks.[27] Judgment and care were apportioned accordingly. Those who were sick and poor might merit charity, or they might merit punishment, depending on whether they were viewed as being innocent or at fault. Poverty was no longer an unfortunate state that merited help from the lucky; instead, as one historian of the period explains, it had become "a moral condition to be evaluated and judged."[28]

Who was easier to judge than the pox-ridden poor? Already suspect, the poor were seen as idlers, wastrels, or worse; those with syphilis bore the signs of their vices on their suppurating bodies. It was better for all concerned simply to exclude them from care. Many people felt that there was no good reason to shelter and feed these dangerous and wicked sinners, and, often enough, institutions and municipalities acted according to these beliefs.

DOCTORS, PATIENTS, AND EXPECTATIONS

How did the treatment of syphilis square with the social and medical expectations of the time? How did it relate to the diseases that had gone before, and what kind of model did it provide for those to come?

These are not easy questions to answer. Even at the beginning of the twenty-first century, the study of "outcomes evaluation" is still a new and uncertain part of health care management; for times long past, standards and results are even more difficult to evaluate. Still, we have enough information to gain insights into what people expected medicine to accomplish in these centuries, and to evaluate whether syphilis was handled appropriately for the standards of the day.

Compared to today, people in Renaissance Europe expected relatively little of medicine. They saw health and illness, explains medical historian Katharine Park, not as polar opposites, but as variable points along a continuum. Moving patients from one point on this scale to another at which they felt more comfortable was probably seen as successful treatment by patient and practitioner alike. Probably few people expected to live lives free of pain and suffering; if physicians, surgeons, and herbalists could free them from their more acute and pressing problems, patients probably felt they had been treated properly.

Still, many were discontented with those who provided health care—particularly with physicians, who were often seen as arrogant and grasping. When epidemics struck, people looked to medical men for protection, but they were usually disappointed in the results. Even in 1370, for example, plague prompted the Italian humanist Francis Petrarch (1304–1374) to send the following accusation to a professor of medicine: "Doctors promote themselves shamelessly, making exorbitant claims about their competence. Yet when faced with an emergency like plague, they can only inveigle the trustful out of their money and watch them die." Three centuries later, Thomas Sydenham (1624–1689), the "English Hippocrates," admitted that many poor people were alive precisely because they could not afford to pay for medical treatment. As time went on, hopes rose higher, but this often led to greater disappointments. One eighteenth-century French doctor wrote that he could handle the expectations of the general public. He complained, however, that "what is annoying about the upper classes is that, when they come to be sick, they absolutely want their doctors to cure them."[29]

Treatments for syphilis provoked similar reactions, as von Hutten's bitter recriminations about mercury plainly showed. The punitive harshness of syphilis treatments, combined with the expense and the judgmental attitudes with which medical authorities commonly administered them, speaks ill of the times, as does the expulsion of the pox-ridden from hospitals, cities, and towns. Physicians and surgeons multiplied the torments of the sick; quacks exploited them for easy cash. Doctors and divines alike reminded the sufferers and their neighbors that the pox was a sign of wickedness. Von Hutten died, penniless and syphilitic, at the age of thirty-five, sheltered by the Swiss reformer Hyldrich Zwingli but rejected by Erasmus, his former friend. Summing up his experiences with the clergy, von Hutten bitterly remarked, "The divines did interpretate this to be the wrath of God, and to be his punishment for our evil living. And so did openly preach, as though they, admitted into that high council of God, had there learned, that men never lived worse." The physical burdens of syphilis were thus made even heavier by social, medical, and moral torment. To a modern viewer, certainly, it seems that the social response to syphilis—like the response to leprosy—revealed not only a failure of health care, but also a failure of the most basic Christian virtue of all, the virtue of charity. Moralizing, for many, took precedence over the fundamental commandments to feed the hungry, clothe the naked, and heal the sick.

Europe was not alone in this regard. Islamic nations judged syphilis as harshly as Christian ones did, just as the faraway societies of East Asia and India had viewed leprosy as divine punishment.[30] The fact that European prejudice against syphilitics was not unique, however, did not make it right—nor did it make it any easier for the rejected to bear.

There were some bright spots in the gloom. Some physicians were moved to compassion for their syphilitic patients. Even the misogynistic Dr. L. S., for example, argued that "the more loathsome the disease, the more commiseration is required, and the physician is obliged to a more tender care." Some cities *were* charitable. Strasbourg opened a special hospital for its syphilitics; Lyon and Frankfurt, soon after the epidemic hit, cut taxes for the sick. The new disease may also have helped to advance medical knowledge and health care, as physicians thought more carefully about infectious diseases, and cities and hospitals developed specialized clinics, rather than treat all the sick poor together in the same infectious wards.

All too often, however, syphilis provoked responses reminiscent of the most brutal and unfeeling reactions to leprosy and plague. Charity and compassion were often overpowered by prejudice and fear. The limits of medical knowledge and old histories of anger and terror at disease proved almost irresistible, and syphilis created even more panic by mixing terror about physical illness with Christian culture's ancient and profound anxieties about sex. Those unfortunate Europeans who suffered from syphilis experienced the worst of disease, medicine, and religious condemnation all at once—a deadly mixture, and a dangerous model for the centuries ahead.

CHAPTER FOUR

A Broom in the Hands of the Almighty:

Bubonic Plague

It is hard to underestimate the fear plague aroused in medieval and early modern Europe. In the face of its epidemic outbreaks, the civil bonds that normally held society together ruptured completely. In the most devastating episodes, such as that of 1348, when a third to a half of the population of Europe and the Middle East died, "brother forsook brother, uncle nephew, sister brother, and oftentimes wife husband," as poet Giovanni Boccaccio (1313–1375) lamented; "fathers and mothers refused to visit or tend their very children, as [if] they had not been theirs." In periods of sickness, populations were so diminished that many a chronicler noted that grass grew in the streets of cities and towns.[1] Through the eight plagues that bore down upon Florence between 1340 and 1427, the city's population shrank to one quarter of its former size, and those few who remained huddled together in an oversized and empty urban shell.[2]

The symptoms of the disease were terrifying: the infected were tormented with painful boils "the size of an apple or an egg"; they coughed until they could not breathe; they vomited green and black fluids, or even pure blood. They lost consciousness. Their eyelids turned blue, their faces the color of lead, their eyes red and swollen. Had the disease not been fatal, perhaps these "signs" or "tokens" might have troubled the victims less, but in fact the death sentence was swift and sure. Most of those who fell sick died, and died quickly. If infected by the bites of rat-borne fleas, or by breathing in bacteria spewed into the air by a coughing sufferer, people died from plague within a few days. Those infected by blood-to-blood contact died within a few hours—often with no warning symptoms at all. And before the days of antibiotics, the mortality rate of plague ranged up to 90 percent. In plague time, the average medieval life span dropped almost by half, from something over thirty years to something under twenty. Premodern remedies were completely ineffectual; prevention efforts, as Katharine Park has noted, were as futile as they were aggressive. In the period when it stalked the Continent, from the sixth century to the eighteenth, plague was the deadliest disease Europe knew. The only effective way to avoid this hasty, painful, and ugly death was to flee before the onslaught.[3]

Unlike the afflictions examined in other chapters of this book, plague was not specifically tied to transgressions involving sex. It was so strongly associated with sins of other kinds, however, that it offers invaluable lessons in the history of the idea that disease was a punishment from God. This association found some of its most striking and eloquent expression in the sermons and pamphlets of seventeenth-century English Protestants, such as the one that described plague as "a broom in the hands of the Almighty, with which he sweepeth the most nasty and uncomely corners of the universe."[4] An examination of these fierce but sometimes poetic views will form the culmination of this chapter.

The rhetoric of sin and blame gathered strength from three main sources. One was the increasing centrality of the idea of sin in the stringent moral climate of Europe during and after the Reformation. Another was the continuing closeness between religion and medicine and the increasing gap between traditional medicine and the progress of science, a gap that left medicine unable to meet the growing expectations people had for it. And the last was the increasing presence of, and a corresponding revulsion for, the poor—the most common victims of the disease. All these together made it easy to view the devastating waves of plague not as strictly natural phenomena, but as supernatural punishments visited upon those people viewed as sinful in the eyes of God.

New Ideas Denounced

Scientific knowledge grew enormously in early modern Europe. In 1512, Nicholas Copernicus proposed the idea that the planets revolved around the sun—an idea so radical that it was not accepted until Galileo proved it in 1632.[5] In 1513, Andreas Vesalius moved anatomy forward with his hugely influential book *The Structure of the Human Body*.

The new and disturbing idea that the blood circulated throughout the body was proposed, to little notice, by Michael Servetus, who was born in 1511 and burned at the stake in Geneva in 1554 for criticizing Calvin's theology.[6] Only when William Harvey published *The Motion of the Heart* in 1628 did this theory gain popular attention, and even then it was accepted with great reluctance, since it clearly showed that the old physiology and anatomy were profoundly inaccurate, and suggested that the entire Galenic system, the basis of traditional medicine, was wrong.[7] The seventeenth century also witnessed the popularization of Arabic numerals, the decimal system, slide rules, surveying and navigational instruments, trigonometry, logarithms, double-entry bookkeeping, and tables for calculating rates of interest.[8] Last but not least, in the 1670s Anton van Leeuwenhoeck invented a lens that could magnify minuscule objects up to three hundred times—an invention that would lead to the discovery of tiny organisms living in drops of water—a discovery that would one day change medical science.

For the most part, however, the medical profession turned its back on these revolutionary developments. Medicine continued to be dominated by physicians, who were distinguished from the rabble of other health-care providers—surgeons, midwives, herbalists, religious healers, and even witches[9]—by an intensely traditional training. Medical schools relied on the second-century theories and writings of Claudius Galen until the 1700s, refusing admission to new subjects, approaches, and knowledge. Not only was it conservative; medical education was also hugely time-intensive, and extraordinarily costly as well. To become a physician in seventeenth-century England a man had to have a four-year liberal arts degree, a master's (which could require up to seven years of additional study), foreign medical training, and preparation for a career in the church or civil service as well. And to win entry into the prestigious College of Physicians, home of the profession's leading lights, he also needed a doctorate in medicine, four years of practical experience, and a passing grade in a four-part Galen exam.[10] Needless to say, this lengthy process of indoctrination did not create openminded and innovative practitioners. Most seventeenth-century French doctors, for example, reviled Harvey's theories about the circulatory system as "paradoxical, useless, false, impossible, absurd, and harmful," as medical historian François Lebrun recalls.[11]

Contagion was not an unknown concept in this day and age, but it was still poorly understood, and frequently the measures recommended to avoid spreading the plague from one person to another were misguided or even counterproductive. Some sixteenth-century writers, for example, claimed that the epidemic was spread by "immoderate sexual intercourse"; the London city council in the 1580s was convinced that putting on plays in times of plague would "draw the plague by offending of God."[12] The infected rich remained at home, quarantined with large signs that invoked the mercy of God. These measures may have made the healthy feel better, but they did nothing for the sick and little to protect the public health: the greatest risk of plague came not from human-to-human transmission but from what French historian Emmanuel LeRoy Ladurie has called the "ménage à quatre" of human, rat, bacterium, and flea. Meanwhile, the sick poor were locked away in understaffed, overcrowded, and deadly plague hospitals. Sometimes dogs and cats were killed in an effort to prevent the spread of disease, but this approach merely permitted rats and their infectious parasites to run free.[13]

THE THRIFTLESS POOR

Run free they did—especially in the decrepit, unsanitary, and crowded neighborhoods of the poor, who were by far the most common victims of plague. A sixteenth-century Italian chronicler sniffed that, in one outbreak of plague, all twenty thousand who died were "low people."[14] The English writer Thomas Vincent, too, remarked that while the rich and middle classes had left London, "the poor are forced (by poverty) to stay and abide the storm." Sometimes this fact inspired pity and charity among those with means, but often it inspired revulsion and fear: those who had been spared frequently convinced themselves that others had perished because they deserved to die. The targets of this prejudice varied with the times. In the Middle Ages, in outbreaks of plague, Christians had burned to the ground hundreds of Jewish communities from Catalonia to Germany, often with their residents trapped inside. In seventeenth-century England, people frequently assumed—and announced—that those stricken by plague had been taken for their sins. And often the crime of those who were struck down, according to the survivors, was simply the fact of being poor.

The poor occupied a somewhat different place in post-Reformation Europe than they had in earlier centuries, and this new position left them more open to blame. Economic life was harsher, and so more people lived on the edge of disaster. Difficult climatic conditions contributed to poor harvests and a general lack of food; prices consistently rose faster than wages.[15] With hunger, overcrowding, dirt, and disease their constant companions, the poor were almost always sick, and most of the sick were poor.[16]

Plague turned these hard times into catastrophes. Spain was visited by the disease in 1599, Switzerland in 1610 and 1615, the Netherlands in 1623–1624 and 1634–1635, northern Italy in 1630 and 1656–1657. The century's greatest epidemic began in Turkey in 1661 and reached Europe in successive summers, attacking the Netherlands in 1663 and London in 1665 before heading east again. As plague decimated the indigent, the rich often reviled them for having brought their disease upon themselves; and when this deadly and unpredictable disease escaped its "natural" social boundaries, the rich, as plague historian Paul Slack has observed, blamed their sick and dirty neighbors all the more.[17]

A SPECIAL OR SPIRITUAL MEDICINE FOR THIS TIME OF INFECTION OR ANY OTHER TIME

Without an accurate theory of contagion, physicians had little to offer in the way of prevention advice except the old and accurate adage *cito, longe, tarde:* Flee quickly; go far; return late. As for explanations, medical authorities threw up their hands. Some physicians followed classical beliefs and blamed the stars; others argued that the problem was religious, not scientific, and left the question of origins to the divines, "because it exceedeth the bounds of Nature." More often, people believed that mysteries like plague showed the interdependence of the doctor and the priest or minister; such an attitude made sense in the views of an age in which no great chasm separated religion and medicine. What varied among physicians, in fact, was not whether they turned to religion in their quest to understand disease, but whether their religious views inclined to charity or condemnation. As with syphilis, some doctors sought to heal those afflicted with plague, while others judged them and found them guilty as punished. The same was true of divines. Some, like Luther, argued that as God had brought diseases into the world, so had he provided humankind with remedies in the form of medicine and doctors. Others took a more fatalistic view. For them, humanity was sinful, punishment and suffering were inevitable, and the only appropriate response was to accept these evils and see in them the will of a just and fearsome God.

Increasing, and increasingly suspect, poverty; a revived emphasis on human sinfulness; reconfigured notions of charity—all these, combined with repeated onslaughts of a terrifying and deadly disease that medicine could neither prevent nor cure, meant that people needed some way to understand and cope with what was happening to them. Certainly not all of Reformation Europe took an identical view of the relationship between religion and medicine, disease and sin, but within the spectrum of opinions certain trends emerged.

Some were quite pragmatic. Luther, for example, announced that people should fight and avoid disease whenever they could. In an essay entitled "Whether One May Flee from a Deadly Plague," he argued that it was pointless and even sinful simply to accept all of life's catastrophes as God's punishment. Those who turned away from apothecaries and physicians, or lingered needlessly in cities as the epidemic bore down on them, were as foolish, Luther stated, as those who refused to flee a burning house or refused to pray to escape the torments of heaven. All these ills came from God, but people nevertheless had the responsibility of avoiding them when they could. "God created medicines and provided us with intelligence to guard and take good care of the body so that we can live in good health," he explained. To do anything else would be to become "a suicide in God's eyes." Christians, Luther urged, should provide hospitals and nursing care for the sick, but quarantine and even flight were appropriate preventive measures. Preserving health through earthly means was not only legitimate for Christians—it was required of them.[18]

Laurent Joubert (1529–1583), physician to the kings of France and Navarre and chancellor of the Montpellier medical school, voiced the same opinions. Quoting the book of Ecclesiasticus in his work entitled *Popular Errors concerning Medicine and a Healthy Lifestyle,* Joubert advised the sick to reconcile themselves to God—and then to consult the doctors, whom God had created and to whom he had given medical knowledge. It was up to the theologians, Joubert suggested, to feed the soul with piety and water it with holy doctrine. The physician, on the other hand, should restrict himself to his vocation: "to care for the human body, keep it in health, and restore it to health when it has fallen away."[19] The priest had one job, Joubert argued, and the doctor another; while they might well be complementary, they were not the same.

This, however, was not the only point of view. According to some thinkers, the physical and spiritual were not separate; disease was simply God's punishment for sin, and the only legitimate and effective source of cure was not medicine but religion. These sentiments were widely shared. Catholic theologians in late seventeenth- and early eighteenth-century France, for example, explained that disease was to be welcomed as a divine corrective that "afflicts the body but contributes to the heal-

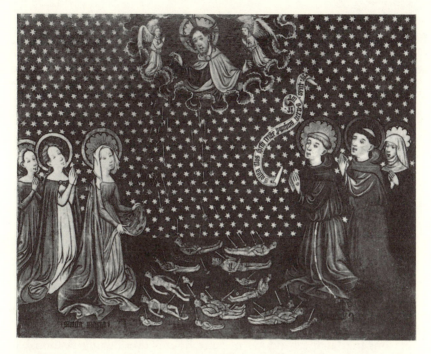

Christ Hurling the Arrows of Plague. Anonymous. Painting on wood, on the altar of the Barefoot Carmelites, Göttingen, 1424. Courtesy of the Wellcome Trust Medical Photographic Library, London.

ing of the soul," mortifying the physical self to render it obedient to the spirit. And a citizen of Marseilles, writing in the middle of the great plague of 1720 which killed half of his city's inhabitants, wrote that the epidemic "seems to serve only to show that all human industry and aid can do nothing against the severity of an angered God."[20]

This view was strikingly expressed in the many religio-medical writings on plague of seventeenth-century England, an age in which traveling from religion to medicine required no great leap.[21] What varied was not so much whether physicians and divines believed that God had a hand in healing, but the view that members of both professions took of God and man. For some, God was a generous and compassionate spirit, extending help to humanity in times of trouble. For others, people were almost irredeemably sinful, punishment and suffering were inevitable, and the only appropriate response was to accept these evils and see in them the will of an angry, righteous, and fearsome God. Both these attitudes—and many degrees in between—were found in the extensive literature on plague, and both would influence attitudes toward disease both in their own day and in the centuries to come.

TEARFUL BODINGS OF A DESOLATING JUDGMENT

"Shall a trumpet be blown in the City, and the people not be afraid? Shall there be evil in the City, and the Lord hath not done it?" With these words from the book of Amos, Thomas Vincent began his 1667 pamphlet *God's Terrible Voice in the City*, in which he told the dreadful story of the London plague of 1665.[22] Plague had struck Holland in 1664, and by the following May, its first fearsome signs were seen in the English capital. In the first week of the month nine people died of plague in London and its suburbs, an "arrow of warning," in Vincent's view. The following week, the death toll dropped to three; fears were banished as people took hope that the city might be spared. But the next week, the figure rose to 14, then to 17, and then to 42. "Now secure sinners begin to be startled," Thomas observed; "now a great consternation seizeth upon most persons, and tearful bodings of a desolating judgment." Fear had alighted in Londoners' breasts, and with that fear came the guilt of those conscious of their sin.

Bit by bit, people began to leave the city. First to depart were the upper classes: suddenly few rustling gallants walked the streets, few ladies lingered at the windows of large houses overlooking fashionable squares. As the gentry cowered in the relative safety of their country retreats, the bills of mortality sounded louder and louder alarms to those who remained in town. In June the weekly count rose to 112, then 168, then 267, then 470: God was warning people to prepare themselves. Sweet roses withered in garden and market as people armed themselves against infection with the bitter odors of wormwood and rue. Meanwhile, another kind of bitterness stalked the streets, as the sick were sealed up in their houses behind the armed guard of warning signs and quarantine. "It was very dismal," Vincent recalled, "to behold the red crosses and read in great letters LORD HAVE MERCY UPON US on the doors, and watchmen standing before them with halberds." These houses stood so solitary, and people passed them with such fear, that it seemed as if the streets were lined with enemies lying in ambush.

In July, as Vincent chronicled, plague poured over the walls of the city like the waters of a flood. Higher and higher rose the piles of the dead: 725 one week, 1,089 the next, then 1,843, then 2,010. The piles of coffins terrified people in the streets; infected houses received no visitor save a nurse, while lovers, friends, companions stood aloof. Convinced their days were at an end, the living saw before them "the grave . . . now opening its mouth to receive their bodies, and hell opening its mouth to receive their souls."

Still there was no abatement in the black tide: in August, the weekly mortalities rose from 2,010 to 2,817, to 3,880, to 4,237, to 6,102. For Vincent and his contemporaries, these were the days of the apocalypse. "Now death rides triumphantly upon his pale horse through our streets, and breaks into every house almost, where any inhabitants are to be found. Now people fall as thick as leaves from the trees in autumn, when they are shaken by a mighty wind." The city grew silent as a Sabbath day: shops shut, no horses or carriages abroad, none of the famous cries of London's street hawkers. "If any voice be heard, it is the groans of dying persons, breathing forth their last, and the funeral knells of them that are ready to be carried to their graves."

Vincent described pitiable and horrifying tableaux: a mother carrying her child's little coffin to bury it with her own hands; a man, demented with plague, who smashed his face against a wall until he was laid under a tree to die; another—sick, lonely, and distraught—who set himself on fire in his bed. And still the death toll mounted: in September, it rose to 6,988, and then fell briefly to 6,544, raising hopes that the epidemic would pass with the approach of autumn. The following week, however, it climbed to 7,165. At this moment, all hope was lost.

For Thomas Vincent and many of his peers, the catastrophe showed clearly that the citizens of London had sinned, and that for this reason God was casting torment down upon their heads. Even those who sought to escape in revelry and sensual delights could not persist in their denial; in the foxholes of the plague, there were none who did not believe. This ravaging epidemic, it was clear to all, was the handiwork of the Lord. The churches were so full that ministers could not pass through the aisles, and were forced to make their way to their pulpits by clambering over the pews. Never had they had so rapt an audience; every eye, ear, and heart was open to the word of God.

Even in this field of converts and believers, however, diverse opinions bloomed. To some, plague was a just punishment that made the wicked suffer and sacrificed their wayward lives. Others, however—like Vincent—noted that "this disease makes little discrimination, and not a few fearing God are cut off amongst the rest. They die of the same distemper with the most profane, they are buried in the same grave, and there sleep together till the morning of the resurrection." Plague took saints and sinners together in its rapacious grasp. How were people to understand this tragedy, and what did their religion have to teach them about it? This was the quandary to which Thomas Vincent and his fellow divines were called.

Seventeenth-century England was full of writings that straddled the border between theology and medicine. Books and pamphlets with names like *Medicines for the Plague* and *The King's Medicine ... Prescribed by the Whole College of Spiritual Physicians* offered religious advice, not physic.[23] They were not supplements to medical care, but substitutes for it. Referring to the familiar adage on how to prevent plague, one author wrote that "bodily physicians" recommended physical flight: "Depart speedily, far off, and return slowly." This "spiritual physician of our souls," however, had a more sovereign prescription, "a better flight": he advised his readers to run "to the name of Jehovah ... by the feet of prayer."[24]

The cause of all physical illness, these spiritual physicians averred, was the evil actions of humankind. And if sin was the cause of sickness, as the anonymous *London's Lamentation* (1641) assured its readers, it was equally clear that "the best means to procure health and safety" must be prayer. Presenting prayer as "A special or spiritual medicine for this time of infection or any other time," *London's Lamentation* recommended preventive doses both morning and night. There was no mistaking why people were beset with disease: "[God's] sword is drawn against us, and what is the cause? Alas, it is the multitude of our sins." The failings of humanity were many and great. "We cannot say," the author admitted, "that thou dost use any injustice in punishing us for our sins [which] cry loud in thy ears for vengeance"; only divine mercy could abate the righteous punishment humanity had merited. This mercy had but one remedy: Christ, who had been sacrificed on the cross to take away the sins of the world. "Let his crimson blood wash away our scarlet sins," this fearful author begged his readers to pray.[25] For him and all who shared his beliefs, sin was the clear cause of plague, and prayer and repentance its only cure. John Donne (1572–1631), poet and dean of St. Paul's, voiced the thoughts of many when he wrote,

> When plague, which is thine Angel, reigns,
> Or wars, thy champions, sway,
> When heresy, thy second deluge, gains;
> In th' hour of death, th' eve of the Last Judgment Day,
> Deliver us from the sinister way.[26]

THE LORD WILL FIND THEM OUT

Thomas Vincent's contemporaries shared the view that plague—and disease in general—was a punishment from God, and that humanity had to turn back to God for healing. They tried to carry some message of redemption to their readers. Even so, however, there was a dramatic range of sentiments, from dark recrimination to a warmer gleam of commiseration and hope. For some plague writers, life could best be described in the famous phrase of their contemporary, the philosopher Thomas Hobbes (1588–1679), who saw it as "solitary, poor, nasty, brutish, and short": life's sufferings and disappointments were no surprise to them. Others, however, looked at the same bleak picture and brightened it with words of comfort.

The most somber writers reveled in the sufferings caused by sin. One, Thomas Doolittle, in his 1665 treatise entitled *A Spiritual Antidote against Sinful Contagion in Dying Times,* threatened the wicked that "a dark and stinking grave will be too good a place for the bodies of unpardoned sinners to remain in." Others gave dire warnings too: Edward Lawrence, in *Christ's Power over Bodily Diseases,*[27] cautioned his public that even the gentlest of excesses—even the kindly virtue of parental love—could be punished by dreadful pain. "Sometimes a father is too fond of a child," he noted, "and the very might and strength of his heart, which might be better exercised in the love and service of God of Jesus Christ, is vainly wasted . . . in the inordinate love and delight" he lavishes on his offspring. This attachment to earthly things was anathema to the jealous God in whom Lawrence believed: a God who, sending down disease, "presently leaves a fatherless child, or a childless father." Human suffering was a mere feather in this scale, in which righteousness weighed heavy and mercy light.

Lawrence and his fellows took plague as welcome grist for their theological mill, and any advice physicians could give was trumped by the preachers' card.[28] Doctors might well advise their patients to run from plague, but it was no matter: "so long as they carry their sin with them, the Lord will find them out, and his hand will reach them wheresoever they are." If physicians argued that plague was spread by physical contagion from one body to another, "I. D.," the author of *Salomon's* [i.e., Solomon's] *Pest-House or Towre Royall,* knew better: "If we carry within us the plague of sin, the inward cause of the bodily contagion, we have no warrant to be safeguarded."[29] The body and its ministers could not hold a candle against the ministers of the soul.

These writers read divine meaning into every aspect of human sickness, and their lesson was always the same: that man was sinful, and disease was not a natural phenomenon but the awesome punishment of an angry but righteous God. What was plague? asked Francis Herring (d. 1628). "Not a disease, but a monster, overmatching and quelling ofttimes both Art and Nature, . . . the stroke of God's wrath for the sins of mankind." Diseases, Lawrence preached, were "God's arrows, [which] can only hit us and hurt us when it is God's will to shoot them into our bodies." Herring and Lawrence were not shy to embrace this somber theological view which, as theologian Karen Armstrong points out, turned God into a "cruel and despotic tyrant."[30] "We shall never be sick till our Father be willing to make us sick," Lawrence asserted, taking as a point of doctrine that "all sicknesses and disease are at the will, and under the command and government of Jesus Christ." It was true that "inferior causes," such as poor diet and the seasons of the year, might open men's bodies to disease; ultimately, however, God was the "first and chiefest cause."[31]

Lawrence did try to deliver a modicum of hope along with his dire tidings: all human suffering, he explained, served to bring people closer to their maker. The consolations he offered, however, were harsh and frightening. "As the fire melts and softens the gold, and thereby fits it for the stamp," he reasoned, "so these sicknesses soften the hearts of the godly, and thereby fit them to receive the stamp of God's image." Believers must remember that life was a sacrifice, prepared for God and "to be always ready to be offered to him at his will and pleasure." Those who sowed in tears would reap in joy, he assured them in the words of the Psalms, but for the most part the tears were in the present and the joy only a wan promise for some far-off future day. More dismal attempts at reassurance could be found in Lawrence's reminder of all the "millions of diseases" and "mountains of torments" that God kept from his worshipers every day, but these ideas could hardly have brought much happiness to those whose loved ones had been wrenched from them and who feared that they might wake up on any morning covered with the black and swollen signs of their own mortality.

The most severe of the English plague writers saw little joy in life, and the destruction wrought by plague gave them a chance to broadcast this fire-and-brimstone message to all who would listen to their sermons or read their words. Their primary purpose was to remind men and women of the evil in their hearts and natures, and to warn them that it was their responsibility to avoid incurring God's wrath. "When thou art tempted to any sin," Lawrence admonished, "remember thy sickness: consider, wilt thou bring again upon thyself an ague, fever, dropsy, consumption, etc.?" In an era wracked by plague, it did not take much imagination to see what this ominous "et cetera" might be. Prayer was the only preventive these preachers could offer—prayer and repentance. And when all else failed and death descended, perhaps some comfort could be gleaned from the familiar Pauline adage that *Salomon's*

Pest-House recalled: "While we are in the body, we are absent from home."[32]

THE FALLOW GROUND OF OUR HEARTS

A slightly less gloomy and more compassionate view of the sufferings of plague was offered by Thomas Swadlin (1600–1670), author of *Sermons, Meditations, and Prayers upon the Plague*.[33] Swadlin had no question about why God had sent such pestilence down upon London: it had come "because we are sinners, because we are great sinners," he declaimed. And the sins of London must have been grave indeed, he argued: ordinary sins begot ordinary diseases, "but the desolation of pestilence never followed unless some great abomination preceded." He cited "barbarous lusts" among his fellows, such as polygamy and incest, but ultimately no member of the populace was exempt from wrong. "All of us are sinners, all."

Swadlin's iconography of suffering was as harsh as any plague writer's, but he always took care to make his images serve some higher purpose: divine affliction, no matter how great, would bring redemption in the end. God's punishment was simply "physic," Swadlin reasoned. The Lord hurt only in order to heal. If people would listen to words, God would have no need of blows; if he did send a plague, it was with great reluctance. "He would fain lay aside this sharp plough, but he cannot otherwise break up the fallow ground of our hearts," Swadlin explained. "Fain would he lay aside these hammers, but he cannot by the instrument of words beat understanding into our brains." If God punished his creatures with pestilence and death, he did it because nothing else could save them.

Swadlin knew of physical medicine, of course, but he gave it little credit. The only relevance it had to his sermon on plague was to provide a rich vein of imagery, and often these images reflected the most violent practices of the physician, the apothecary, and the surgeon—practices that made the cure as frightening as the disease.

> So long as God punishes you, he gives you physic. If he draw his knife, it is but to prune you; you are his vine. If he draw blood, it is but to rectify a distempered vein: you are his patient. If he break your bones, it is but to set them straighter. If he bruise you in mortar, it is but that you breathe up a sweet savor into his nostrils: you are his handiwork. And if one hand be under you, let him lay the other as heavy as he pleases upon you. Let him handle you which way he will; if he does not throw you out of his hands, it is no matter.

The scenes Swadlin created in the minds of his congregants were violent ones, if undergirded by a notion of paternal, corrective love.

Love was, in fact, the deepest foundation of Swadlin's *Sermon*, and if it was harsh and cruel at times, he nevertheless took pains to show that it was there. God directed his anger and punishments only toward his friends, Swadlin insisted: "The father whips his own child, not his neighbor's, or a stranger's. Nor doth *God* whip another people, but his own." The faithful could take comfort in the fact that, if they suffered, it was only because God desperately wanted them to know he cared, and to turn them toward him and away from sin. One critical aspect of Swadlin's sermon was that he warned his readers to avoid a grave error of interpretation: if plagues came from God with love, it meant that those afflicted were God's creatures above all. "You that love," he cautioned, "must take heed how you censure them that die: for the plague, to die of the plague, is no evidence of reprobation."[34] In a tract full of suffering and sin, this author could not fail to remind his fellow Christians that one of their greatest duties was compassion toward those on whom God had lain the heavy hand of correction.

An even broader compassion was shown by Thomas Vincent in *God's Terrible Voice in the City*. Rare but poignant among texts of this kind was the personal note Vincent sounded: unlike many of his contemporary preachers, Vincent depicted himself among the suffering and the fearful victims of plague. One short passage in particular brought home the devastation wrought by the epidemic—a passage which foreshadowed the losses that would be brought to America and the world three centuries later by AIDS.

> Now the plague had broken in much amongst my acquaintance, and of about sixteen or more whose faces I used to see every day in our house, within a little while I could find but four or six of them alive. Scarcely a day passed over my head for I think a month or more altogether, but I should hear of the death of some one or more that I knew. The first day [I would hear] that they were smitten; the next day some hopes of recovery; and the third day that they were dead.

Perhaps such losses taught Vincent to look at the question of sin differently than many of his contemporaries. Most striking among the catalogue of London's sins he enumerated were the failings of the pious, such as hypocrisy in the profession of religion, formality and lukewarmness in the worship of God, the deafening of the ear against God's call, unmercifulness, and the perversion of judgment. Even more striking, in looking down the list of sinners and their sins, Vincent wrote that he would prefer "to begin here with myself," and urged readers that any who found parallels in their own consciences should "consider and lay to heart" the experience and advice he offered. Sin, for Vincent, might well be the cause of plague, but rather than blame others, he advised all who would listen carefully to examine themselves.

MOVED BY THE ANGEL

Historians record that many, even most, people in the seventeenth century viewed disease as a natural phenomenon—a normal and more or less inevitable part of life. Plague, however, was an exception. "It was the haphazard incidence of plague," explains Paul Slack, "which more than anything else proved its divine origin. The way in which it hit one house and not another, one town and not another, could be explained only by the hand of God." If plague swept away the wicked, they were being punished; if it reaped the lives of the just, they were being brought to their reward. Plague was so devastating and so overwhelming that it could be understood only by ascribing it to divine intent, no matter how mysterious that might be.[35]

Divine intent, of course, was always read through human eyes, and these readings varied according to how the interpreters viewed the world. Some, as we have seen, were almost savage, and could be bitterly cruel. In 1563, the English town of Dartmouth, as a preventive measure, expelled all its sick poor in one wretched heap. In the following decades, English plague victims were abandoned in the streets and left to die and be eaten by dogs and pigs, while in 1666 the English government decreed that the bodies of those who had died of plague could not be buried in ordinary churchyards. Expelled from society in life by their sickness, the victims of plague were permanently banned from the community in death.[36] This extreme level of revulsion and fear paralleled the fearsome rituals to which medieval society had subjected lepers and Jews, and foreshadowed the cruelest recriminations twentieth-century American fundamentalist ministers would issue about people with AIDS.

But the mystery of God's will inherent in plague left room also for more generous and compassionate responses as well. In Renaissance Florence, many citizens were moved to care for the plague-stricken poor out of a concern that repeated onslaughts of disease were God's way of condemning the community for being uncharitable.[37] In England, Swadlin reminded his readers that they had a duty to be loving toward the sick; Vincent reminded his readers that the pious were sinners, as well as the profane. Plague may have provoked the Christian reader to point a finger at others' sins, but at least some of the time it also prompted him to ponder the book of his own heart.[38]

In the autumn of 1665, the London death-toll finally began to subside. From its high-water mark of 7,155, the black tide of weekly mortality ebbed to 5,538 at the end of September. Within five weeks it had dropped to 1,031, and by the end of November it had fallen to 333. The total number of those lost to plague in this fearsome year was 68,596, as against only 6 the year before. The deadly lesson had redeemed some of his fellow citizens, Vincent gratefully recorded: "Now the net is cast, and many fishes are taken; the pool is moved by the Angel, and many leprous spirits and sin-sick souls are cured." Some of these died of the plague in peaceful acceptance, like the teenaged boy in Vincent's household for whom faith and hopes of martyrdom removed the sting and fear of death. Others survived and continued to walk steadfast in the paths of virtue. Vincent lamented, however, that those whose sudden conversions had been motivated only by fear "with the dog returned to their vomit, and with the sow have wallowed again in the mire of their former sins. . . . They that were drunken are drunken still, . . . they that were unjust and covetous do still persevere in their sinful course . . . as if there were no significance in God's judgments by the plague." This return to normalcy was quickly ruptured by the Great Fire of London the following year, but even those scars on the face of the city gradually healed, and saint and sinner began their lives again.

Both social and religious responses to plague, from the Middle Ages to the seventeenth century, showed a range of values that comprised the worst and the best in human nature. Like leprosy, syphilis, and other epidemics that were still to come, plague inspired pity and terror, accusation and kindness, charity and fear. Some of these responses were universal, while others varied with religion, time, and place, but all formed part of a long tradition of human efforts to understand the terrifying destruction epidemics could wreak on human life.[39]

Like leprosy, plague gradually faded out of sight in Europe after the great epidemic of 1720 in Marseilles. With it, too, passed the powerful assumption that religion and medicine were inseparably linked. With the advent of the Enlightenment, the balance of power between science and theology shifted, and most people began to take substantially different views of the phenomena of the physical world.

A striking feature of the history of medicine, however, was that—

especially for diseases linked with sex—many old attitudes about sickness and sin continued to thrive even after this cultural revolution took place. The following chapter, on the medical treatment of masturbation, shows how these attitudes made an extraordinary leap from the chapel to the consulting room in the case of a behavior that might never have been viewed as a sickness had it not first been seen as a sin.

CHAPTER FIVE

The Heinous Sin of Self-Pollution:
Medicine, Morals, and Masturbation

Even as plague faded away, Europe—and the European colonies in the New World—became traumatized by the fear of a new phenomenon that they were convinced gave rise to an almost endless number of physical, psychological, and moral evils. The medical establishment claimed that masturbation led to deadly symptoms that ranged from lassitude to consumption (tuberculosis), blocked or burning urine, stupidity, paralysis, spontaneous gangrene, apoplexy, and even death. After having been diagnosed with masturbatory insanity, men and women by the dozen were locked away in mental asylums. Patients reported that they had eaten ground glass and locked themselves into suits of armor to restrain themselves from the dreaded habit. Physicians prescribed hydrochloric acid, strychnine, and belladonna to cure the evil, and they performed brutal operations—cauterization, clitoridectomy, circumcision, and even castration (sometimes with anesthesia, sometimes without)—to keep their patients from practicing "self-abuse."

Awaiting anyone who sank to these depths was not only devastating harm, but also utter moral ruin. Health-food pioneer and Seventh-Day Adventist John Harvey Kellogg, M.D. (1852–1943), inventor of the cornflake that bears his name, warned that "the most loathsome reptile, rolling in the slush and slime of its stagnant pool, would not bemean itself" by masturbating. With few exceptions, the entire medical establishment of his day agreed with him. What was behind this collective delusion?

THEOLOGY AND MEDICINE

For centuries, theologians had condemned masturbation, while medical authorities paid it little attention. (Galen had simply noted that Diogenes the Cynic masturbated as a quick and easy way to rid himself of the nuisance of sexual desire: "If only I could remedy hunger by rubbing my hand on my belly!" the philosopher had lamented.) Around 1700, however, the concept of "self-abuse" leapt over the dividing line between religion and medicine, as doctors warned for the first time that masturbators were endangering not only their souls, but their bodies as well. The medical response passed through several stages. At first, doctors trumpeted warnings; then, late in the eighteenth century, they began to prescribe drugs to combat the effects of this vice. The nineteenth century endorsed preventive and corrective surgery, the twentieth the psychiatrist's couch. Throughout this process, one common theme emerged: in an increasingly scientific and skeptical age, the doctor assumed the role of the priest. In accepting this power, however, the medical profession did not create a new set of moral values; instead, it largely accepted the old view—that health was morality and morality health. The sacraments of confession, penance, absolution, and redemption were now administered by the physician, rather than by his ecclesiastical brother.

Even today, when official silence on the subject reigns in the American Psychiatric Association's *Diagnostic and Statistical Manual of Mental Disorders,* popular attitudes reveal that masturbation still provokes embarrassment, guilt, and nervous laughter; Americans teasingly warn one another that solitary sexual indulgence will cause blindness, acne, or sweaty palms. Psychological and sociological surveys reveal that, for reasons they do not entirely understand, 50 percent of Americans still feel guilty about masturbating. Few know that the old wives' tales they joke about were the medical dogma of an earlier era, and that their guilt and anxiety have a long and honorable pedigree.

The reasons for this fear of masturbation were many and complicated. Some were tied to religious dogma that saw any sex unredeemed by procreation as a sin. Some were social: the changing conditions of European life may have made it easier for young people to masturbate in their newly private beds and bedrooms than to engage in premarital sex. And others were medical. The symptoms of masturbation were confused with those of gonorrhea and syphilis; symptoms of mental ill-ness were taken for cause. And once demonized, masturbation served as a convenient culprit for ills physicians could diagnose but not cure. All this weighed heavily on the medical profession and its patients alike.

Like the seventeenth-century English preachers who denounced the plague-ridden for their sins, nineteenth-century physicians condemned the immorality of those they believed were sick with a new disease. Like the Renaissance doctors who tortured syphilitic patients with mercury and cautery irons, their later counterparts poisoned and burned the bodies of those who practiced "self-abuse." There is no question that these doctors thought they were acting in the best interests of their patients, but there is also no question that patients were severely hurt—even when they willingly agreed to their torture. Ultimately, the medi-cal treatment of masturbation was a grievous error based on faulty as-sumptions and dangerous logic. How people made this mistake, and where it took them, is the story of this chapter—the story of how medi-cine, morality, and masturbation became intertwined.

Dangerous Pollutions

Masturbation had long troubled the consciences of the pious. St. Au-gustine and other early Christians believed that involuntary sexual fan-tasies were caused by demons who took over the human mind and memory to lead their unfortunate victims down the hellish paths of sin; medieval Jewish and Christian sages alike feared that ejaculated semen would breed devils; medieval Catholic evening prayers besought God to keep the supplicants chaste and pure throughout the night.[1] Illusion and pollution—mental desire and its physical expression—entangled soul and body in a dangerous and sticky web.

The Bible gave these theologians reason to worry. They found a model for masturbators in Onan, a character from the book of Genesis. When his brother died, Onan was required by Hebrew law to carry on the dead man's line by making his widow pregnant. Onan started to follow the law's command, but then had a change of heart: he inter-rupted the coitus, "spilled his seed upon the ground"—and was imme-diately struck dead by God.

On first blush, the story of Onan does not seem to be about mastur-bation. Theologians, however, found a common element in coitus inter-ruptus, masturbation, anal intercourse, and other kinds of nonmarital, nonvaginal sex acts, which they judged to be unredeemed by pregnancy and procreation. All of these were bad, but masturbation inspired a special fear in the hierarchy of the Catholic Church, since it represented a purely physical act of sex, unredeemed by even the possibility of procreation—and also since it could be performed even by monks in the isolation of their cells. What could be more of a threat to men and women sworn to celibacy than the haunting desires that came from deep within their minds and turned them toward secret, illicit, and lustful action? It was scarcely surprising that, in the early Middle Ages, prayers and books of penance should have besought God to restore to purity "anything polluted through negligence, or committed by anger, or stimulated by drunkenness, or subverted by passion," as a tenth-century German service instructed bishops to pray.[2]

As the centuries passed, this fear became a panic, and none panicked more than the eminent reformer and educator Jean Gerson (1363–1429). One might imagine that Gerson had more important things to do than worry about masturbation: among other weighty responsibilities, he served as chancellor of the University of Paris, and also helped resolve the ecclesiastical crisis known as the Great Schism, in which two and then three simultaneous claimants to the papacy struggled with one another for power. Despite the weight of these administrative and political burdens, however, Gerson found the time to write not one but two treatises on this "abominable and unnatural" vice.

These treatises sent priests on an elaborate fishing expedition into the consciences of the guilty parties. Clearly, even six centuries ago Catholics felt guilty about masturbating, and it was up to their confessors to find their way past the lay people's defenses. Greet your subject familiarly and affably, Gerson's treatise advised its priestly readers, counseling them not to be too direct, but instead to descend by degrees, almost obliquely, to their true subject. "Friend," the priest should casually inquire, "do you remember [handling your erect penis] when you were around ten or twelve years old? It is well known that all boys do this." Bait the hook with kindness and sympathy, Chancellor Gerson suggested: do not let the man think that what you are asking about is dishonorable or shameful. But, once he is hooked, reel him in hard. If he tries to escape by retracting what he has said, remind him that lying in the confessional—lying to God!—is the gravest sin he can commit. Do not let him get away, because, once caught, the penitent can be saved by prayer, prescriptions for abstinence, holy water, and absolution; only then can he be released. As a final measure, the anxious Gerson provided a special form of absolution for monks, prime targets of the solitary vice.[3]

Gerson set the tone for later churchmen, who continued to worry that even the purest souls could fall to perdition at any time. A seventeenth-century catechism, for example, taught the faithful how to guard themselves against temptation when they were lying in bed, awake and exposed to sin. Immediately upon awakening, it urged them to lift their hearts up to God, make the sign of the cross, dress promptly and modestly, and pray; the goal was to pass through the dawn without being tempted. In the perilous evening, the reins were pulled yet tighter. Pray again at bedtime, the watchful catechism advised the faithful; examine your conscience; make confession. Then undress in silence, make the sign of the cross with holy water, and go modestly to bed. Until you fall asleep, the book grimly advised, you must think of death, eternal repose, and the sepulcher of Our Lord.[4] This tense and gloomy nighttime ritual left no room for minds or hands to do the devil's work.

Doctors, before 1700, rarely worried about self-stimulation as such; what they did worry about was whether their patients were properly regulating the flow of sperm. With semen as with everything else, the medical doctrine of the humors taught that excessive depletion was as dangerous as the extreme abstinence that caused lovesickness. The second-century physician Aretaeus the Cappadocian, for example, warned that even young patients who lost too much seed "necessarily became old in constitution, torpid, relaxed, spiritless, timid, stupid, enfeebled, shriveled, inactive, pale, whitish, effeminate. . . . For it is the semen when possessed of vitality, which makes us to be men, hot, well braced in limbs, hairy, well voiced, spirited, strong to think and to act."[5] To lose semen was to lose what made men men.

At the heart of this concern, however, was a crucial ambiguity. Men could lose sperm in a number of ways, the ancient physicians believed. Excessive sexual intercourse was one; nocturnal emission (and perhaps masturbation) was another. But equally dangerous was what the Greek doctors called "gonorrhea" ("flow of seed"). For centuries, priests and physicians did not clearly distinguish the venereal disease we now know by that name from the spontaneous nocturnal emissions experienced by postpubescent males who have no other sexual release. This confusion, joined with a tradition of moral anxiety, led the medical profession to lump venereal disease and masturbation into one single pathology until the twentieth century.

The conservative training of seventeenth- and eighteenth-century physicians encouraged them to follow their predecessors in the area of seminal loss as in all others. Writing on the maladies of women in 1587, the French doctor Jean Liébault warned that seminal losses could lead to paralysis and convulsions, and recommended purges and vomits as a cure. Nicolas Venette (1633–1698), who taught the mysteries of sex to much of Europe in his book *The Picture of Conjugal Love,* warned against excess too. Sexual overindulgence, Venette cautioned, dried up the brain and caused asthma, fever, liver problems, sterility, and gout. Even these alarms, however, were sounded not against masturbation per se, but against undue loss of semen through any means. Like all good Galenic physicians, Venette warned against not only excessive sex but also excessive abstinence; the same was true of the wildly popular sex guide *Aristotle's Master-Piece,* which ran through at least forty-three editions between 1684 and 1800. But masturbation, narrowly defined, had not yet really emerged into medical consciousness as a separate area of concern.

WOMEN AND CHILDREN

The eighteenth century saw a number of conflicting trends with regard to sex. On the one hand, a certain sexual license prevailed, especially among the higher social classes in France, as witnessed by such literary works as Choderlos de Laclos's *Dangerous Liaisons* (*Les liaisons dangereuses,* 1782) and the novels of the Marquis de Sade (1740–1814). Men still retained substantial sexual freedoms: condoms (made of animal gut or oiled silk) came into use in the eighteenth century, for example,[6] and men who patronized prostitutes were protected by the medical and legal establishment, which argued that these clients were only following the call of nature. Elsewhere, however, morality was becoming stricter. Social rules placed women under the control of men, as the eminent Philadelphia physician Benjamin Rush explained in a letter to his fiancée: "Don't be offended when I say that from the day you marry you must have no will of your own. The subordination of your sex to ours is enforced by nature, by reason, and by revelation."[7]

One area in which nature, reason, and revelation bore heavily down on women was in bed. Women who refused to be sexually docile and socially subordinate were viewed as unnatural and dangerous—"monsters in human shape," as Dr. M. T. D. de Bienville explained in his book *Nymphomania* (1775). Overwhelmed by uterine fury, Bienville wrote, these deranged women would sexually assault men, and, when appropriately rejected, would often indulge their vengeance in the perpetration of "the most cruel and tragical crimes." To cure his unnatural patients, Bienville placed them in restraints for months at a time, and injected potent drugs into their vaginas—injections, the doctor confided, these women were eager to receive. Eighteenth-century medicine went to great lengths to keep men on top.

Women were not the only people who had to stay in their assigned place; children did too. As infant mortality rates gradually declined, parents' attitudes toward their children subtly changed. Families became more encompassing and more corrective, and formal education taught children their proper roles in society. Toilet training was harsh, and whipping became more common among many, while fathers and mothers with strong Protestant convictions schooled their children less by beating than by fierce instruction in the code of conscience and shame. "Break [your child's will] now," advised John Wesley (1703–1791), the founder of Methodism, "and his soul shall live, and he will probably bless you to all eternity."[8] The new propriety's viselike grip affected children's sexuality as well. In earlier years, children had treated their bodies more freely—the childhood physician of Louis XIII of France (1601–1643), for example, recorded how the young prince cheerfully displayed his juvenile member to the royal household.[9] In the eighteenth and nineteenth centuries, however, these free and open attitudes gave way to stringent and repressive moral control. One of the aspects of adolescent life that would come to be governed most harshly was sex, and medicine proved to be a highly effective means of enforcement.

PHYSICIANS ABOUNDING

Eighteenth-century medicine helped to maintain the new propriety. The medical profession was becoming more scientific; it was also growing more expansive, claiming title to new domains. With the approval of an increasingly rationalistic society, physicians legislated right and wrong by declaring some things healthy and others diseased. Though more ambitious than ever before, however, the medical profession's reach still exceeded its grasp; in England in 1700, one infant in three died before the age of five, and the average life expectancy was only thirty-seven years. People remained suspicious of doctors: as the English magazine the *Spectator* announced, "When a nation abounds in physicians, it grows thin of people."[10]

In many ways, the suspicions were justified: to a modern eye, eighteenth-century medicine seems a strange hodgepodge of science and nonsense, as seen in the recommendations of self-help books such as Wesley's *Primitive Physick* (1747, reprinted in 142 editions until

1871), "The Angel of Bethesda" (1724), written by New England Puritan leader Cotton Mather (1663–1728), and Dr. William Buchan's *Domestic Medicine* (1769). Wesley recommended drinking cold water (alone or mixed with sulfuric acid) to cure plague; a live puppy held constantly on the belly, he asserted, would remedy colic. Mather prescribed powdered alum dissolved in red wine for diabetes, "a bit of Negroes' wool in the ears" against deafness, and hogs' dung mixed with nettle juice—taken externally *and* internally—for greensickness, a disease of young women that had elements of medieval lovesickness and anemia combined. Dr. Buchan warned that people who cogitated excessively "generally become quite stupid" and rarely lived to be old.[11]

Along with this advice, however, these men also offered insights and suggestions that modern readers would readily approve. They were quite interested in Anton van Leeuwenhoeck's 1674 discovery of "animalcules," for example. Declaring these tiny organisms responsible for smallpox, Mather championed inoculation, a practice recently imported from Africa and Turkey, and saved many lives in the process. He warned, too, against smoking and snuff. Wesley proposed twice-daily gargles with salt water to kill the germs that give rise to gum decay; Buchan urged frequent hand-washing, and noted the connection between heavy metals and occupational diseases in mercury miners, plumbers, painters, and gilders. He was also deeply concerned with improving children's health.

Yet with all these advances, the old links between sickness and sin remained strong; if anything, in fact, these connections were reinforced by the rise of Puritanism. Mather, for example, told women that they should blame their gynecological problems on Eve. "Think: the sin of thy mother, which is also my sin, hath brought all this upon me!" For Wesley, the best preventive was still the love of God, since only this "effectively prevents all the bodily disorders the passions introduce." Childhood illness was particularly troubling for religious parents, who often felt that their children were suffering for their own sins.[12]

All these developments came together around the beginning of the eighteenth century, and masturbation was a critical point of focus. It unified new and old religious concerns, and gave physicians entrée into a new area—sexuality—that was closely related to the developing fields of gynecology and pediatrics. Additionally, for a medical profession that was increasingly able to recognize problems it could not yet cure, self-abuse was an easy culprit to link with all kinds of diseases nobody could otherwise explain. Turning masturbation from a religious problem into a medical one filled a long list of unmet needs, both social and scientific.

FAR BELOW THE BRUTE CREATION

The transformation began with a few texts of dubious medical standing. In a 1697 Latin tract against fornication, an obscure author named Adriaan Beverland warned that self-abuse was both sinful and—what was new—suicidal. Whoever spilled the precious oil of semen, Beverland cautioned, raised violent hands against himself: "Idleness leads to lust, lust to disease, and disease to untimely death." This dire chain of causality was taken up by one physician after another, and the focus on masturbation grew sharper and sharper.

The next voice to cry out was that of an anonymous Englishman, perhaps clerically trained, who had a sharp ear for new and powerful ideas and a product to sell. Around 1715, this author published a pamphlet entitled *Onania, or, the Heinous Sin of Self-Pollution, and All Its Frightful Consequences, in Both Sexes, Considered.* Dozens of English editions followed; American versions appeared starting in 1724; German translations sold hundreds of thousands of copies. *Onania* spread to its avid readers the terrifying news that to ejaculate without intercourse would cause stunted growth, disorders of the penis and testes, gonorrhea, epilepsy, hysteria, consumption, and barrenness. Finally, following the biblical example from which it took its name, *Onania* warned that the vicious would meet their deaths.

Effective countermeasures were essential, the pamphlet advised. A male sufferer could tie his penis to his neck with a string, for example, to prevent erections and ejaculations during sleep. Marriage was another good preventive; so were cold bathing and a milk diet. But the best remedies of all were the "Strengthening Tincture" and "Prolifick Powder" for sale by a certain London merchant at ten and twelve shillings the box. All of *Onania*'s dire warnings, it turned out, were a means to peddle a product—one of the many over-the-counter drugs whose advertisements filled the newspapers of the Georgian age.

Onania was tremendously successful at alarming the public. Not only did thousands of readers buy the pamphlet (and, no doubt, the powders it promoted), but many other authors began to pick up on what was clearly becoming a popular obsession. One of these followers was an eminent Swiss doctor, Samuel-Auguste-André-David Tissot (1728–1797). By giving onanism credibility as an official medical problem, Tissot changed the history of masturbation forever. *Onania* may have been popular, but it had few claims to intellectual respectability; Tissot, on the other hand, published widely, corresponded with Voltaire and Rousseau, and was physician to a pope. When Dr. Tissot added a treatise on the evils of masturbation to his 1758 dissertation on malaria, the educated classes of Europe paid close and continued attention. His treatise saw sixty-three editions and thirty-four translations into five languages, and remained in print until 1905.

In language that mixed the authority of medicine with the power of religion, Tissot showed in graphic and gruesome case studies how self-abuse sent many young people into moral and physical decline. Tissot wrote that his patients died in despair, the mouth of hell gaping around them, and described them as criminals whom their suffering chastised for their dreadful crime. One particular invalid was the picture of disso-lution by the time the doctor arrived at his bedside. As Tissot drew him, this man had been reduced by masturbation to

> a being that less resembled a living creature than a corpse. . . . A watery, palish blood issued from his nose; slaver constantly flowed from his mouth. Having diarrhea, he voided his excrement in bed without knowing it. He had a continual flux of semen. . . . The disorder of his mind was equal to that of his body. . . . Far below the brute creation, he was a specta-cle, the horrible sight of which cannot be conceived, and it was difficult to discover that he had formerly been part of the human race.

THE LAWS OF NATURE

Such fearsome warnings as this set European medical circles ablaze with anxiety. Eager to capture and distribute the latest and best infor-mation on all subjects, people turned to Tissot for whatever news they could get about this dreadful and newly identified scourge. Among these researchers were the philosopher Denis Diderot and the mathe-matician Jean d'Alembert, editors of the *Encyclopédie, or Reasoned Dic-tionary of Sciences, Arts, and Trades*, first published from 1751 to 1765. In seventeen volumes of articles and eleven more of illustrations, Did-erot and d'Alembert preached a new gospel of scientific enlightenment. Severely censored and very nearly suppressed by the Jesuits and the French Council of State, the *Encyclopédie* was the master text of the French Enlightenment: what it said, the new and influential intelligent-sia trusted and believed. In a series of articles on masturbation and re-lated topics, the *Encyclopédie* endowed the ideas of Dr. Tissot with a philosophical respectability that lasted throughout the late eighteenth and nineteenth centuries.

In a way, masturbation was the perfect subject for the *Encyclopédie*. Diderot and d'Alembert leavened their secular learning with a nonsec-

tarian morality based on Judeo-Christian values and what they saw as
the fundamental principles of nature. Both science and morality condemned masturbation, Tissot had argued, and the authors of the *Encyclopédie* agreed. Onan, they explained, had deprived his sister-in-law
of the opportunity to become a mother, and so God deprived him of
his life. Those who followed his example broke the social bond with
their "criminal hands," wasting the precious fluid that had been designed to perpetuate the human race. This suicidal practice, the Ency-
clopedists noted, caused self-abusers to die in the profoundest sorrow
and regret. Their death was nothing but the vengeance of an outraged
Nature who "has no shortage of tortures to cause expiation of the crimes
committed against her laws. She adjusts their violence to the gravity of
the harm." The diseases that masturbation caused were no more than
nature's rightful due.

Thinking like this made sense in the eighteenth century, the Age of
Reason, which believed that physical phenomena and human morality
were based on the inviolable principles of "natural law." These ideas
found expression in the American Declaration of Independence (1776),
which cited "The Laws of Nature and of Nature's God" to justify its
solemn pronouncements, and in the French Revolution as well. The
new medical and moral views of masturbation aligned comfortably with
these principles—especially so when they had been officially approved
by Tissot and Diderot, and then endorsed by such eminent and pro-
gressive thinkers as Jean-Jacques Rousseau (1712–1778) and Voltaire
(1694–1778).[13] Fears and worries about masturbation carried not only
the old burden of thousands of years of religious prohibitions, but also
the new weight of medical and scientific proof; modern ideas about social propriety and increasing concerns about children's and adolescents'
health added yet more power. The fit between old and new values was
too good, the reasoning too compelling to ignore; by the end of the
eighteenth century, most of Europe and much of America were thoroughly terrorized by the horrific dangers of self-abuse.

Le Mal du Siècle

If anything, the nineteenth century was even more preoccupied by masturbation panic than the eighteenth had been. Fears spread from the
medical profession to the general public, and people worried not only
about their bodies, but also about their minds. These increased concerns summoned graver treatments. While earlier writers had mostly

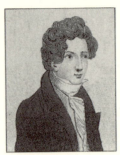

Il était jeune, beau :
il faisait l'espoir
de sa mère...

He was young and
handsome—his mother's
hope...

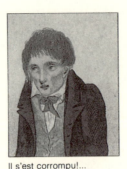

Il s'est corrompu!...
bientôt il porte la peine
de sa faute vieux avant
l'âge... son dos
se courbe...

He became corrupted!
Soon his crime makes
him old before his time.
His back becomes hunched.

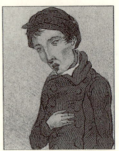

Un feu dévorant embrâse
ses entrailles; il souffre
d'horribles douleurs
d'estomac...

A devouring fire burns
up his entrails; he suffers
from horrible stomach
pains.

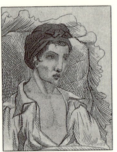

Voyez ces yeux naguères
si purs, si brillants,
ils sont éteints! une bande
de feu les entoure.

See his eyes, once so
pure, so brilliant: their
gleam is gone! A band
of fire surrounds them.

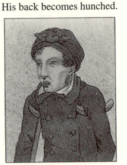

Il ne peut plus marcher...
ses jambes fléchissent...

He can no longer walk;
his legs give way.

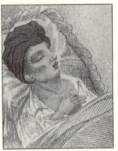

Des songes affreux
agitent son sommeil...
il ne peut dormir...

Dreadful dreams disturb
his rest; he cannot sleep.

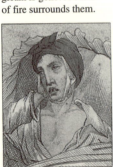

Ses dents se gâtent
et tombent...

His teeth become rotten
and fall out.

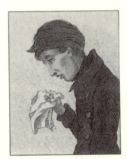

Sa poitrine s'enflamme..
il crache le sang...

His chest is burning up.
He coughs up blood.

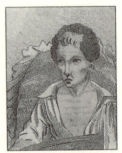

Ses cheveux, si beaux,
tombent comme dans
la vieillesse; sa tête
se dépouille avant l'âge...

His hair, once so beautiful,
is falling out like an old
man's; early in life, he is
becoming bald.

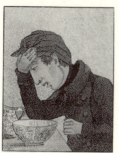

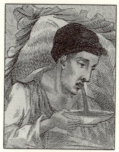

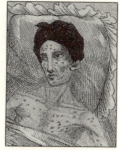

Il a faim; il veut apaiser sa faim; les aliments ne peuvent séjourner dans son estomac...

Sa poitrine s'affaisse... il vômit le sang...

Tout son corps se couvre de pustules... il est horrible à voir!

He is hungry, and wants to eat; no food will stay in his stomach.

His chest is buckling. He vomits blood.

His entire body is covered with pustules; he is a horrible sight!

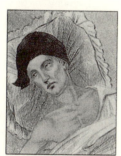

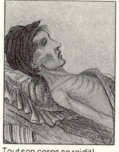

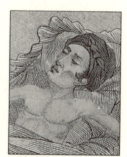

Une fièvre lente le consume, il languit : tout son corps brûle...

Tout son corps se roidit!... ses membres cessent d'agir...

Il délire; il se roidit contre la mort; la mort est plus forte...

A slow fever consumes him. He languishes; his entire body is burning up.

His body is becoming completely stiff! His limbs stop moving.

He raves; he stiffens in anticipation of coming death.

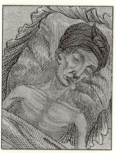

A 17 ans, il expire, et dans des tourments horribles.

At the age of 17, he expires in horrible torments.

"The Fatal Consequences of Masturbation." From *Le livre sans titre* (The book with no title), 2nd ed. (Paris, 1844).

called for moral suasion to prevent and correct the solitary vice, physicians in the new century increasingly turned to straitjackets, harsh chemical preparations, cautery, and the knife.[14]

This anxiety was closely linked to the nineteenth century's tormented ambivalence about sex. Sex was part of love and marriage, the cultural ideals around which young women of the era planned their lives, but it was kept far out of the public eye, immured in the fortress of privacy known as the home. As social historian Michelle Perrot explains in *A History of Private Life*, the home was

> protected by walls, servants, and darkness. . . . The arrangement of rooms for various uses, the location of stairways and corridors . . . were governed by strategies of encounter and avoidance. . . . Household sounds were an amalgam of cries and whispers, muffled laughter and sobbing, murmurs, surreptitious footsteps, squeaking doors, and the implacable tick of the clock. At the center of all this secrecy was sex.[15]

Inside marriage and outside of it, discomfort about sex governed much of nineteenth-century life in Europe and America. People worried about the risks posed by naked bodies—even their own. Mid-nineteenth-century medical surveys, for example, found that many French people feared that an hour in the bathtub might lead them down dangerous paths; many people (especially women) had never washed their bodies from head to toe.[16] Adolescent sexuality troubled these anxious folk too, and so physicians sought ways to delay the onset of puberty. The Catholic Church championed the Virgin Mary as a model for all women: the Immaculate Conception became official dogma in 1854.

Doctors debated how much sex was healthy, or even whether sex was necessary at all. They recommended that patients restrict themselves to one act of intercourse per week (and that, naturally, within the confines of marriage). Over-frequent sex was viewed as horrendously dangerous; so was sex late in life (i.e., past forty-five for women, fifty for men). John Harvey Kellogg warned Americans that reckless indulgence of this kind invited "disease, premature decay, . . . and running the risk of sudden death: Nature cannot be abused with impunity." Any kind of sexual excess, including masturbation, called for the most drastic of corrective measures, warned Samuel Bayard Woodward, writing in 1835 that *"Nothing short of total abstinence from the practice can save those who have become the victims of it."*[17]

Yet the prudish Victorians, who squirmed at the indecency of exposed piano legs, were profoundly hypocritical as well. Enormous numbers of women who had not found their way into marriages sought the harsh refuge of prostitution and the streets. Venereal disease was rampant, and to protect themselves against it, men wore condoms of vulcanized rubber produced in great quantities in Charles Goodyear's factories from the 1870s on.

If these protections were manufactured only for men, it was because only men were supposed to want sex. "As a general rule," explained the Paris-trained English urologist William Acton (d. 1875), "a modest woman seldom desires any gratification for herself. She submits to her husband's embraces, but principally to gratify him; and were it not for the desire of maternity, would far rather be relieved of his attentions." More assertive women frightened authorities social, civil, and medical. French suffragist Hubertine Auclert (1848–1914), opined a police report, "is believed to be suffering from madness and hysteria, a disease that causes her to look upon men as her equals."[18] Women who transgressed the proscribed sexual boundaries were actively forced back behind the lines. In fact, argues cultural scholar Eve Sedgwick, gynecology and psychiatry were developed in good part as the medical profession looked for new ways to control female self-abuse.

This interest in sexuality was typical of the nineteenth-century medical profession, which continued to broaden its scope. Some of the developments were concrete. Effective and reliable anesthesia was developed in the 1840s, and antisepsis two decades later; these techniques alone reduced postsurgery death rates by as much as two-thirds. Life expectancies increased, as well. At the beginning of the nineteenth century, in France, people could expect to live only to the age of thirty; by 1913, however, French men could look forward to an additional eighteen years of living, and French women to twenty-two. Public health and hygiene were clearly making a difference.

The Reverend Doctor

Equally striking were changes in the ways the medical profession saw itself. What had been an art and a craft was becoming a priesthood: as the influence of the clergy declined, physicians more and more took over their role as guardians of specialized knowledge, professional secrets, and philanthropic benevolence.[19] In 1826, Baron Cuvier sang the praises of the physician to the French Chamber of Peers. It was the doctor, he announced, who had "plumbed the depths of the greatest problems of human nature, the heart and body of man. He must rise to every height of the metaphysics . . . of soul and body. He must understand all the innermost resources and bizarre turns of the heart." Less rhapsodic but more concise, Parisian novelist and gadfly Barbey d'Aurevilly (1808–1889) noted that "in a society that is becoming more and more materialistic, the confessor is the physician."[20] In 1868, a French doctor correspondingly observed that to specialize in public health and hygiene was to be "a professor of morals."[21]

The doctor's office replaced the confessional booth—particularly in matters of sex. As German homeopathic physician Wilhelm Gollmann insisted in 1855, "The first duty of the physician consists in obtaining from the patient a confession of his errors, and a firm promise that he will abandon his evil practices. Until this is done no treatment can be of any avail. . . . The ruinous consequences of self-abuse must be continually kept fresh in his soul's memory."

Masturbation became an increasingly pressing source of concern in the nineteenth century, particularly for those people whom society considered incompetent to take care of themselves: children, women, and the mentally ill. Immature, feeble, fragmented, and volatile, members of these groups were ideal subjects for a medical profession seeking to expand its power by enforcing social norms.

Children in particular were a source of constant worry. Long before Freud, masturbation had raised the specter of childhood sexuality, which was by definition a sexuality out of control. Jean Gerson had warned in the fifteenth century that masturbation was especially common among the young. So had *Onania* and Dr. Tissot, whose arguments were especially persuasive, explains critic Ludmilla Jordanova, because he gave medical credibility to old fears about children and sex.[22]

NAMBY-PAMBY MOLLYCODDLES

The telltale evidence of masturbation, physicians and the public believed, was easy to spot in the altered appearance and character of the young people who practiced it, no matter how hard they tried to keep their vice a secret. The faces of the guilty became pale, their eyes sunken, their hands clammy and moist. As medical historian Robert H. MacDonald points out, a poster boy of this unsavory type was the writhing, self-abasing character Uriah Heep in Charles Dickens's 1850 novel *David Copperfield*. When young Copperfield first encountered Heep, he saw a cadaverous face belonging to "a red-haired person—a youth of fifteen, as I take it now, but looking much older . . . who had hardly any eyebrows, and no eyelashes [and] a long, lank skeleton hand [that] felt like a fish in the dark." These repugnant physical attributes were generally joined to an equally slimy character. Cold and callous, masturbators were commonly judged incapable of generosity, loyalty, altruism, industry, honesty, or love.

Masturbation ruined boys' and girls' characters in opposite ways. Boys were at risk because the secret vice attacked the masculine fiber that entitled them to their dominant role in society. Physician William Acton explained that the adolescent most at risk was not the strong, vigorous, athletic young man, but instead "your puny exotic, whose intellectual education has been fostered at the expense of his physical development." The secret vice attacked weak, effeminate, and unmanly boys, and made them weaker still. Masturbating girls, on the other hand, risked acquiring an aggressive and unwholesome masculinity.

Even as late as 1915, fears about masturbation and manliness persisted. In the years just before America entered World War I, John Wanamaker's Philadelphia department store distributed to its teenaged male employees a booklet entitled *The Strength of Ten: What Manhood Is, and How a Boy May Win It.* Its author, Winfield Scott Hall, held impressive credentials. Armed with M.D. degrees from both Northwestern University and the University of Leipzig, Hall taught biology at Haverford College and at Northwestern; he gave U.S. Public Health Service–sponsored lectures at military schools, academies, and colleges, and served as president of the Child Conservation League. This formidable savant was deeply concerned with preserving the vigor of the American male. Healthy boys, Hall told his audiences, were full of "spermin," a substance "carried to the muscles in a thrilling, throbbing stream," making them "bigger and bigger and harder and harder" as the boy approached the full glory of manhood. Hall asked his boy reader whether he would prefer to grow up to be a simpering gelding or a gallant stallion, a beast whose "masculine shoulders, massive hips, and swelling muscles stood for unlimited power." Continent boys could attain this triumph, Hall asserted, but masturbators never would. Instead, self-abusers could only expect to grow into "slope-shouldered, narrow-chested, flabby-muscled, beardless, squeaky-voiced, namby-pamby mollycoddles, . . . cringing, cowardly, docile beasts of burden, useful as slaves, but useless as men."

How to prevent this crisis of masculinity? All authorities agreed: children had to be kept, as Acton put it, in "perfect freedom from, and, indeed, total ignorance of, any sexual affection." They had to be kept separate from one another, too, because the threats of masturbation and homosexuality were often intertwined. Boarding schools must avoid at all costs the dangers of the double bed and of boys' "fashionable" crushes on one another. Above all, boys were not to be left to their own devices: the vice president of the French Anatomical Society, for example, was in favor of conducting regular surprise inspections of the young. The war had to be waged on every available front to protect young men from losing their manhood to themselves or to one another.

Just as it made men less manly, masturbation made women less feminine. Women who stimulated themselves without the aid of a man could become obsessed with sex and thus unfit for their proper role in society. For this reason, athletic practices like horseback riding were to be eschewed; so too were pedal-operated sewing machines, which could stimulate working women until they became sexually sick. The bicycle, another newfangled contraption, also raised alarm, reported an article in the *American Journal of Obstetrics* in 1895. "In France and Chicago the number of women who ride bicycles is said to be large; in Brooklyn their numbers are increasing rapidly, and the exercise, in contagious form, is reported to be spreading even in New York." The author of this article, Robert Latou Dickinson (1861–1950), one of the foremost gynecologists of his day, hastened to assure his readers that, with occasional exceptions, the benefits of cycling outweighed its risks, but he was far from insensitive to his colleagues' fears of what he referred to as the "horrible habit" of masturbation.[23] As Wilhelm Gollmann explained, masturbation in females provoked a wide range of disorders: "Headache, depression of spirits, obstinacy, sadness and indifference to worldly pleasures, and, finally, melancholy and other forms of mental derangement" could all result from the vice. Masturbating girls ran the risk of becoming "tribades" who parodied the sexual behavior of men.

One of the darker fears that troubled physician and public alike was sexual and gender perversion. Just like the modern "sick" homosexual, notes critic Paula Bennett, masturbators were seen as narcissistic and unnatural. In light of these fears, it is hardly surprising that many physicians tried hard to normalize their masturbating patients. Some followed their medieval predecessors and recommended sexual intercourse as a cure for the dysfunction, though others worried that this plan was fruitless. Repeatedly, however, the patients doctors pronounced "cured" were those who conformed to social codes by marrying and having children. These actions proved that they were no longer sexual renegades, and that the "professors of morals" had succeeded in their self-appointed task.

ASYLUMS, DRUGS, DEVICES, AND THE KNIFE

Those who could not fit into the nineteenth century's proper social roles were often defined as mentally ill, masturbators among them. Tissot had associated onanism with various nervous disorders, a link that was confirmed by the famous Philadelphia physician Benjamin Rush, who announced that "chronic aberrations frequently have been found in the cerebellum of onanists." Many others followed, explaining that masturbation was not only dangerous, but addictive as well. T. de Bienville, M.D., noted in 1775 that the habit encroached imperceptibly over the self-control of the "wretched criminal."[24] Léopold Deslandes, M.D. (1797–1852, a member of the Royal Academy of Medicine in Paris), ominously concurred: "When onanism once commences, it is difficult to say how far it will extend."[25]

To control onanists, and to keep them from troubling society, physicians—and their families—often kept them under lock and key. Of the patients admitted to the French asylum of Charenton between 1825 and 1833, forty-four men and three women were diagnosed as insane because of "libertinism or onanism." Of the 272 mentally ill patients admitted to the Paris hospitals of Bicêtre and the Salpêtrière during the same period, forty-one men and eighteen women were onanists. Boston physician Samuel Woodward said in 1835 that approximately 10 percent of the male lunatics he had observed had lost their reason through masturbation. Ten percent was a relatively low estimate, in fact: the superintendent of the Massachusetts State Lunatic Asylum reported to his state legislature in 1848 that a full 32 percent of his inpatients had gone mad from self-pollution. This figure was soon quoted far and wide, and set the tone for medical views of the age, in which doctors described masturbation as "a habit which is both ridiculous and vile," as "disgusting and reprehensible," and even as "moral leprosy." Perhaps the echoes of medieval leprosy led doctors to segregate these unfortunates, though it is hard to imagine that the patients' lives were in any way improved by the process.

This undercurrent of moral self-righteousness pervaded many nineteenth-century treatments for masturbation. Some physicians locked masturbators up; others treated them with drugs, physical restraints, the cautery iron, and the knife. Pain and other side effects were no bar to treatment; sometimes they were endorsed and welcomed by physicians and patients alike. One patient of Dr. François Lallemand (1790–1853?), for example, felt that the only way to cure himself of his dangerous vice was to encase his body in a torturous metal garment that rivaled the most extreme forms of medieval self-mortification. Under his clothing, this man wore a twenty-two-pound suit of mail outfitted with a silver basin around his genitals. As a still greater precaution, the patient had sharp points affixed to the inside of the cup. Despite the fact that it damaged his testicles and the spermatic cord, the patient wore this apparatus every day for nine or ten years.[26] No affliction was too painful, no damage too great, because, authorities agreed, no treatment could be more harmful than the vice itself.

Treatment often started from the inside out, with medications that ranged from mild to drastic. Sedatives were commonly prescribed— anything from the run-of-the-mill chloral hydrate and potassium bromide to opium (most effective, Dr. John Laws Milton noted, when mixed into a brandy cocktail). A wide range of homeopathic remedies was available as well. These included the chaste tree (*vitex agnus-castus*, a shrub of the verbena family that had frequently been recommended as a contraceptive by medieval medical writers), marijuana, sulfur, Spanish fly, hot pepper, mercury, strychnine, sulfur, rhododendron, and sea sponge. Nonhomeopathic physicians prescribed such potent substances as ergotamine, digitalis, belladonna, strychnine (which, wrote the ever-helpful Milton, "may be safer and more effective if mixed in very small doses of arsenic"), nitric acid, and hydrochloric acid, of which one source not very reassuringly commented that "a small dose . . . has no appreciable action on the bowels; a larger one purges somewhat freely." Toxicity varied with dosage, of course, but it is hard to believe that these remedies had no ill effects.

Drugs and poisons were one recommended route to health; more direct physical interventions were also freely used. One mid-nineteenth-century New York surgeon, Homer Bostwick, bled his patients by applying leeches to their inner thighs over a vessel of boiling water. (The steam ensured that, when the worms fell away, sated and swollen, the blood would continue to flow.)[27] Other doctors blistered and scalded the penis or perineum of their patients. Others still inserted electrodes into the rectum and urethra, or placed them on the penis in order to pass electrical currents through the body. (Dr. Kellogg recommended using an electrical urethral probe in fifteen-minute doses, two or three times a week.)

These doctors tried to prevent masturbation by stimulating the genitals in painful ways; others tried to prevent sensation, or deaden it. Some put ice on their patients' sexual organs; others administered cold-water enemas. Doctors and parents fastened young infants into straitjackets and chastity belts. Everett Flood, an American physician, wrote an article in 1888 boasting of the success of a plaster cast he had produced to keep a young patient from masturbating: "the boy's genitals might have been in the next county for all the sensation his hands could communicate."[28] Dr. Deslandes, too, was in favor of restraints of all kinds. In boarding schools, he advised, children's hands and feet should be tied up at night. He lauded another physician's device—a "strait-waistcoat, which was laced behind, and was furnished in front with a silver apparatus, to contain the genital organs, and having only an opening for urine." The drawbacks of such contraptions were hardly to be compared with their benefits: though the apparatus might irritate the genitals and their edges cause "deep excoriations . . . they are often useful and ought not to be neglected."

Trusses with silver cups, actually, were among the simpler devices in use. Milton described far more elaborate ones in his book *On Spermatorrhea: Its Pathology, Results, and Complications*, which had gone into its eleventh edition by 1881. Milton recommended the "toothed urethral ring" and the "four-pointed urethral ring," commenting that "the reader must have seen the effects of this little instrument in order to appreciate its value."

Even more startling than these pointed bands was the "electric Alarum." This Rube Goldberg contraption had a ring placed on the penis, "so made, so that when expanded by erection it completes an electric circuit, and so rings a small alarum bell placed under the sleeper's pillow." This system worked quite effectively for several patients, Milton reported. Another, however—a deep sleeper—required that a relative (who, supposedly, "knew nothing of . . . why the alarum was used") stay awake with him all night to interrupt his dreams. "The fifth patient," Milton regretfully concluded, "soon got tired of the alarum" and discontinued its use.

AWAKENED BY PAIN

Some medical men spoke openly about their desire to punish their patients for their immoral behavior, and their surgical practices spoke even more eloquently than their words. None of these procedures was mild. At the least violent end of the spectrum was the very common use of the "bougie," a long, flexible tube of varying thickness made of rubber, metal, or some other material, and inserted into the male urethra. Sometimes bougies were used to clear urinary blockage; sometimes they carried a caustic dose of burnt alum, silver nitrate, or sulfuric, muriatic,

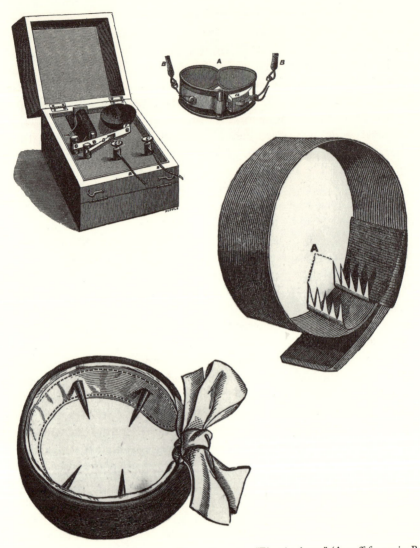

Antimasturbation devices for men and boys. From top: "Electric alarum" (A: cuff for penis; B: leads to alarm box); "toothed urethral ring"; "four-pointed urethral ring," with bow. From J. L. Milton, *Pathology and Treatment of Spermatorrhoea* (London, 1887). Courtesy of the Wellcome Trust Medical Photographic Library, London.

or nitric acid to the opening of the seminal ducts. Whether this chemical cauterization was in itself painful depended on the dosage, but there is no question that the operation itself inflicted trauma on the patients.

Physicians, however, strove to maintain professional detachment. Bostwick, for example, recounted one case in which his probe emerged

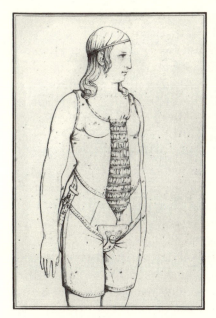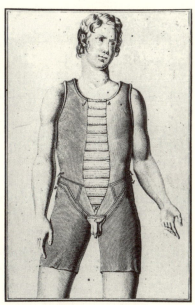

Drawings of antimasturbation trusses (1819). Courtesy of the Wellcome Trust Medical Photographic Library, London.

covered with blood and pus: "The patient fainted while I turned to clean the bougie. [He] fell to the floor, and in the fall struck upon the fender before the fire, and hurt his head considerably." Unfazed, however, the surgeon returned the sound to the urethra and left it in for another quarter of an hour. If a tube could penetrate only with extreme difficulty, Dr. Samuel W. Gross, a president of the Pathological Society of Philadelphia, recommended clearing the way with a knife.[29]

What was not penetrated was often pierced. An ancient practice called "infibulation" (using a pin to fasten the foreskin over the head of the penis) was resurrected in order to prevent erections and seminal losses. Dr. Louis Bauer (1814–1898), a peripatetic surgeon whose career took him from Prussia to London, Manchester, Brooklyn, and ultimately St. Louis, described his technique in 1879. He transfixed the prepuce by two silk slings and directed the patient to tie them together at bedtime. The object of this procedure was "to wake the patient by pain when the penis should get in a state of erection." Bauer was pleased to report that the treatment proved effectual, despite some wear and tear: "The slings, of course, were often renewed at new places in the prepuce as the old ones threatened to cut through." He gave no indication that he anesthetized his patients as he sewed their foreskins up.[30]

Another painful technique physicians recommended—and which male patients sometimes requested—was circumcision. The foreskin, people believed, made masturbation easier and more appealing; removing it was thus a logical step. Did this operation work? Yes, argued Sir Jonathan Hutchinson (1828–1913), a Quaker surgeon who served as Hunterian Professor at the Royal College of Surgeons and as a member of two royal commissions, and was considered to be among the greatest medical geniuses of his day. Hutchinson believed strongly that circumcision helped to keep men chaste. He admitted that it was impossible to be sure of this, since "the distasteful nature of the inquiry" made it impossible to carry out an accurate survey; nevertheless, he was convinced that Jewish men—by definition circumcised—were much less troubled by "the maladies which we associate more or less definitely with masturbation and nocturnal emissions."

In America, Dr. Kellogg, too, favored circumcision, which he specifically urged doctors to perform on small boys. Do not anesthetize them, he wrote, "as the brief pain attending the operation will have a salutary effect on the mind, especially if it be connected with the idea of punishment," as, he underlined, "it may well be in some cases." Not one to single boys out for special treatment, Kellogg also recommended anointing with pure carbolic acid (i.e., phenol, a highly toxic and caustic antiseptic) the clitorises of those females "unable to exercise self-control." Cautery was common, as well, as one of the century's most extraordinary case histories revealed—the story of two young Turkish sisters.

TWO LITTLE GIRLS

In Constantinople, in 1881, a terrified couple called in Dr. Démétrius Alexandre Zambaco to examine their two daughters, aged ten and six—girls who nowadays might be diagnosed as brain-damaged or severely disturbed because of prior abuse. The girls were masturbating obsessively and relentlessly, and their behavior would have shocked any parents—let alone an upper-class Christian Turkish couple in the late nineteenth century. To stimulate herself, the elder daughter rubbed her vulva with any object she could get hold of—sponges, pieces of wood, scissors, forks, hairpins, and worse. The younger daughter—at the age of six—had genital organs "so precociously developed that there are already tufts of hair on the labia majora," noted Dr. Zambaco with alarm. She masturbated as compulsively as her older sister. Perhaps most terrifying of all to their guardians, the girls had taught themselves how to masturbate even when they were imprisoned in straitjackets at night. Constricting their vaginal muscles in such a way as to shake the perineum and make the vulva swell, the girls would lie awake in the silence of a darkened room, producing a muted, rhythmic, sucking sound that struck horror in the hearts of the servants paid to watch them through the night.

Many aspects of this case were deeply disturbing to the doctor. One was the masturbation itself, which the girls carried out even to the point of injuring themselves severely. Describing the six-year-old "little Y," the doctor noted that her sexual organs were inflamed and red as blood, and gave off a thick, nauseating, yellow pus despite several washings a day. Y, he discovered, was lacerating her vagina with a table fork. Another troubling feature of the case was the girls' volatile and antisocial behavior. Ten-year-old "X" was moody, proud, and capricious, and would scratch and bite any child who tried to outshine her in a game. Despite physical restraints, X's deportment in public was so scandalous that people would stop and stare at her in the street. Y would not stop masturbating, even though her parents had her whipped until she was completely bruised. But most dreadful of all was the fact that these girls multiplied their vicious pleasure by sacrilege. X stimulated herself with prayer books, branches from the Palm Sunday service, and, on one alarming occasion, the priest's cassock. Nothing was too sacred to become an accessory in these girls' crimes.

In fact, X did everything she could to offend God, whom she blamed for depriving her of this sweetest of earthly delights. She told the inquisitive doctor that her ambition was to do as much evil as she could, and to this end she called upon the devil. Late one night, X was alone in her bed, and summoned the fiend. "All of a sudden," she confided, "the wardrobe door opened wide and the devil appeared. He was tall and completely black. He made a horrible face. His eyes were green. Then all the wardrobes and dresser drawers opened, and an endless number of little demons came out. It was a horrible sight!" This determination to do ill, perhaps more than any other aspect of the girls' demented behavior, convinced Dr. Zambaco that he had to punish and control them. His urge to do this drove him to lengths as great—and as frightening—as those of his obsessive young patients.

At first, Zambaco administered the standard treatments that had been used against masturbation for more than a hundred years. He bathed the girls in cold water, restricted their diet, and sedated them. He scolded, he reasoned, he chastised, he restrained, he whipped. The results were always the same: nothing could stop the girls from the practice to which they had grown completely addicted. At the end of his resources, the Turkish doctor consulted with an expert in London. For desperate cases, his English colleague advised, an extreme practice was called for: cauterization.

Armed with this advice, Zambaco returned to Constantinople and obtained the parents' consent. Nevertheless, he told the girls he would give them one final chance: if they behaved themselves, he would have no need to bother them. If not, however, "I will be ferociously cruel," he warned. "I will burn your organs with a red-hot iron!" For a few days, the warning worked. Soon, however, the children's good intentions lost out to their compulsion, and at this point the doctor began his experiments with iron, heat, and fear. He recorded,

> On September 11th, in order to frighten her as much as possible, I prepare a display of burning coals. On top of them I place an enormous iron in the shape of an axe. I blow until it turns red. Watching such an infernal scene, the girl trembles. "You didn't keep your promise," I say to her. "I will prove that you were wrong by keeping mine." I show her the big, red-hot iron, but I cauterize her clitoris only with a little stylus, 3 millimeters in diameter, heated red-hot over an alcohol lamp. "If you start again, next time I'll burn you with the big iron, and I will show no mercy."

Improvement followed; then relapse. Five days later, Zambaco cauterized again: three hot points on each of the labia, and another on the clitoris. A large, glowing iron seared the six-year-old girl's buttocks and loins again and again. Ultimately, he noted, the combination of pain and terror did the trick for this child, reducing her voluptuous spasms from forty or fifty a day to a mere three or four. The incorrigible older sister, however, was exiled to the countryside and abandoned to live without the doctor's or her parents' care.[31]

Though the locale was exotic and the treatment severe, Démétrius Zambaco was no tribal shaman or itinerant quack. He had received his medical education in Paris, where he had risen to become the head of a clinic and a laureate of the Academy. The author of eleven books, including a prizewinning volume on syphilis, he returned from Paris to Constantinople in 1872 and practiced there until his death forty years later. His 1882 article "Onanism and Nervous Problems in Two Little Girls" was published in a recognized French medical journal without editorial caveat or comment. And indeed, Zambaco's English colleague Dr. Milton approved of his principles: to cauterize without pain, Milton argued, was an exercise in pointlessness.

BODY PARTS FREELY EXCISED

Cauterization was not the end of this brutal road; some doctors carried corrective surgery further still. Dr. Hutchinson, for example, claimed that "measures more radical than circumcision would, if public opinion permitted their adoption, be a true kindness to many patients of both sexes." Removing the ovaries, the testicles, or even the entire penis, he wrote, might be helpful in subduing unruly sexual desires. But when it came to removing whole organs, controversy raged—just as it does over the traditional African practice of female genital mutilation today.

As early as the 1830s, Deslandes had argued that surgical removal of the clitoris was a promising treatment for girls and women who masturbated. Tracing the history of this operation to Egypt, the Persian Gulf, and central Africa, he suggested that it might serve to "remove in infancy, from the vulva of the girls, certain prominences which, at a later period, might prove inconvenient." The operation, he reassured his readers, "is not very painful—is easily performed. . . . It certainly would not be practiced generally if it caused severe pains, or was followed by bad consequences." Removing the clitoris, he admitted, was a last resort: "But when life is to be saved, or the mind is to be preserved, then we ought not to hesitate." After all, explained this doctor, sexual desires were not strictly necessary for women: even "without these feelings of love, a female may [yet] become a good mother, and a devoted wife."

Deslandes supported his arguments by discussing a case of clitoridectomy performed in Berlin in 1807. A deeply troubled four-year-old girl, he noted, demonstrated increasingly blatant symptoms of idiocy. "Reduced to a state below the brute," this little girl "swallowed her feces, and passed hour after hour in a corner, her tongue lolling from her mouth." By fourteen, she had become a compulsive onanist. Her doctors tried various procedures to break the dreadful habit, including cauterizing her head "to obtain revulsion by the pain." Nothing, however, worked—until finally her clitoris was cut away. "The good effects of the process exceeded all expectations," claimed a triumphant Deslandes. "The disposition to onanism was removed; the mind became expanded; and the education of the patient commenced. In three years, she could talk, read, write, and even play a few tunes on the piano." In exchange for these feminine accomplishments, the loss of a minor and troublesome body part hardly seemed much of a sacrifice.

Despite these apparent successes, however, the practice of clitoridectomy gave rise to a tremendous scandal in England in the 1860s. The case involved a prominent London surgeon, Isaac Baker Brown. Born in 1812 to a well-to-do family, Brown won early distinction at the prestigious Guy's Hospital, and at the age of thirty-five he chose to focus his practice exclusively on gynecological surgery. He helped to found St. Mary's Hospital, and went on from there to build his own hospital for women, the London Surgical Home, where he operated on more than a thousand patients.

Brown pioneered several techniques of gynecological surgery, including ovariotomy, which he believed in so strongly that he performed it on his own sister even after several of his earlier patients had died under his knife. (His sister survived.) Ovaries were not the only female organs Brown believed in removing: he deduced that epilepsy and other nervous disorders were caused by "unnatural irritation of the clitoris." This conclusion reached, his obituary noted, "Mr. Brown immediately set to work to remove the clitoris whenever he had the opportunity of doing so." The patient was sedated with chloroform, and the surgeon proceeded to operate. ("The clitoris is freely excised, either by scissors or knife—I always prefer the scissors," Brown cheerfully explained.) He then bandaged the patient, dosed her rectally with opium, and had her carefully watched so that she would not disturb the dressing and hemorrhage. Following this, the patient, her relatives, and her friends were reeducated in several months of "careful watching and moral training." When this procedure was observed, Brown asserted, patient after patient was "perfectly cured" of her nervous problems.[32]

After a number of such operations, Brown (by then a past president of the Medical Society of London) published a book boasting about his results. His friends had advised against the publication, and they were right: the surgeon and his work were immediately attacked from all quarters. Outraged physicians sent letters to the *Lancet,* and brought charges of quackery and mutilation to the Council of the Obstetrical Society. After a vain defense, Brown was quickly expelled from the Obstetrical Society by a large majority.[33] The record is not clear about why this scandal arose, but it seems possible that Brown offended Victorian society less by his operations than by the fact that he talked so publicly about them. The norms of propriety could not bear being openly flouted.

Almost immediately after his public humiliation, this "generous, hospitable, and kind-hearted man," who had always dressed sprucely in black and worn a flower in his button-hole every day, fell apart. Professionally and financially ruined, he succumbed to illness and "during the last few years of his life was helpless from several paralytic seizures."

Brown died almost penniless in 1873, a cautionary tale showing that clitoridectomy, at least, crossed the line of Victorian medical tolerance.

Male castration also hovered on the boundary between the acceptable and the intolerable. Like Hutchinson, some admitted favoring the practice. An 1865 article in the *Medical and Surgical Reporter,* for example, told of a physician "who had been confined as insane for seven years and who [after his castration] was able to return to practice." In an 1898 report from Texas, a twenty-two-year-old epileptic was sentenced to castration by order of a judge, and with the permission of his exasperated and disgusted father. "The patient was described as facing the operation morosely, 'like a coon in a hollow.'"[34] Often, however, doctors spoke out sharply against removing the testicles. Castration for male sexual disorders, wrote an irate physician in the 1840s, was "as effectual as 'decapitation for inflammation of the brain.'"[35] Fortunately, this wisdom generally prevailed: castration remained an unusual measure, even in an age that approved of medical violence against masturbating patients.

FORBIDDEN BY GOD, DESPISED BY MEN

No rhetoric was too lofty or too melodramatic to express the crime of which physicians accused their masturbating patients. Onanism, vociferated Dr. Milton in his treatise *Spermatorrhea,* was a moral "conflagration," a danger to house and home. The father of English psychiatry, Henry Maudsley, agreed, stating that the masturbator was a criminal whose actions endangered both himself and his neighbors. "The sooner he sinks to his degraded rest," Maudsley concluded sadly, "the better for himself, and the better for the world, which is well rid of him."[36] Borrowing a leaf from the *Encyclopédie,* some physicians spoke of self-abuse as a violation of natural law. Among these were Winfield Scott Hall, advisor to the Boy Scouts, and Dr. Irving Steinhardt, a New York physician who lectured on masturbation to the Emanuel-El Brotherhood and the Educational Society of Brooklyn. "You cannot trifle with Mother Nature and not pay for it," Steinhardt warned his young listeners. "She will punish you every time, and severely enough to make you remember it always." Girls too were at risk. In her 1897 book *What a Young Girl Should Know,* Dr. Mary Wood-Allen of Pittsfield, Massachusetts, called the symptoms of onanism "a very serious penalty to pay for any pleasure that one may derive from this habit."[37]

Beyond the arguments of morality and reason, physicians also reacted to masturbation with plain and simple disgust. Sir James Paget (1814–

1899, considered to be the founder of the science of pathology), for example, did not believe that masturbation was truly more dangerous than other sexual excesses. He regretted this fact, however, wishing that he "could say something worse of so nasty a practice, a filthiness forbidden by God, an uncleanliness despised by men."[38] Dr. Deslandes proposed, as a cautionary measure, that young people be exposed to "the sight of an onanist dying." One of his earlier *confrères*, the French physician and surgeon Marc-Antoine Petit (1766–1811), turned this impulse into an award-winning pastoral poem. The protagonist of *Onan, or, The Tomb of Mount-Cindre*, was a young man who died from the secret vice, despite the love of his father and the prayers of a pious hermit. Petit limned the boy's end as a gruesome warning to his young readers:

> His ulcerated body, wearied by his crimes,
> Multiplied its torments by another hundred times;
> The hungry coffin worm, engaged in dreadful play,
> Came early to its feast, and ate him as its prey.

Americans echoed the disgust in the voices of their continental colleagues. One of the most vociferous was Dr. Kellogg, who devoted a six-hundred-page tome, *Plain Facts for Young and Old* (1886), to the topic of sexual vice. Kellogg spoke of masturbation as the "violation of sexual law," of his being "not more disgusted than shocked," of "loathsome crimes and excesses." He was horrified by tales of nurses who taught infants to masturbate in order to keep them quiet and contented. These women, he averred, could hardly do worse by slitting their charges' throats in cold blood; in fact, Kellogg mused, perhaps outright murder "would have been better." The only thing that could "cleanse the slime from [the masturbator's] putrid soul," he warned, was "one safe, successful weapon: 'the blood of Christ, which cleanseth from all sin.'"

The price of salvation, in Kellogg's eyes, was eternal vigilance against any hints of adolescent sexuality. He listed dozens of suspicious signs to which parents of teenagers should be constantly alert. Failure of mental capacity, love of solitude, mock piety, round shoulders, lack of development of the breasts in females, acne, the use of tobacco, biting the fingernails, unchastity of speech—all were probable indicators that young people were in danger. So were other, more disfiguring, signs. "What Makes Boys Dwarfs?" he asked in his "Chapter for Boys"; "What Makes Idiots?" Girls were told a series of cautionary tales: "A Pitiful Case," "A Mind Dethroned," "A Penitent Victim," "A Ruined Girl."

True feminine virtue, on the other hand, Kellogg portrayed in luscious pink detail, perhaps hoping to increase its allure, or perhaps letting his potent pen get the better of him. "Real girls," wrote this ferocious protector of adolescent morals, "are like the opening buds of beautiful flowers. The beauty and fragrance of the full-blossomed rose scarcely exceeds the delicate loveliness of the swelling bud which shows between the sections of its bursting calyx the crimson petals tightly folded beneath." Kellogg's pink and purple prose may have stretched over swelling desires of his own, but ostensibly, at least, the Midwestern doctor was the sternest of moralists. Like the Church authorities of the Middle Ages, nineteenth-century physicians felt obliged to announce, in increasingly loud and hoarse voices, that nonmarital sex was both harmful and wrong. The transformation of masturbation from a religious to a medical problem had been completed.

SEXUAL FIXATIONS

The twentieth century brought changes to this field, as to many others, but they came only slowly, and met with great resistance at every step. Even the success of psychiatry and psychology served, for decades, simply to transform fears of physical illness into anxieties about mental decay. Only in the 1930s and later did a new openness about sex begin to reduce medical anxieties about masturbation, and, even so, popular attitudes lagged far behind. Guilt about masturbation continues to abound, as does moral condemnation. Even at the very end of the twentieth century, masturbation has become what homosexuality was in the days of Oscar Wilde: self-love that dare not speak its name.

At the turn of the century, Victorian views still ruled the medical and psychiatric roost. In 1893, Sigmund Freud announced that masturbation caused neurasthenia, the weakened and nervous condition that was one of the nineteenth century's most widely diagnosed psychosomatic illnesses.[39] Sexologists Emil Kraepelin and Richard Freiherr von Krafft-Ebing listed masturbation under the heading of Sexual Aberrations, along with exhibitionism, fetishism, masochism, and sadism. And the 1897 edition of a standard pediatrics textbook continued to endorse such ferocious preventive measures as mechanical restraints, corporal punishment, circumcision, cauterization of the clitoris, and blistering of the inner thighs and vulva.[40] Psychologists followed along. G. Stanley Hall, in an influential two-volume study on adolescence, described onanism as "one of the very saddest of all aspects of human weakness and sin."

He blamed it on everything from late rising, to attendance at the theatre, to cocaine, and argued that it harmed its practitioners psychologically, physically, and morally.

This leading psychologist believed that the best way to stop sexual transgressions was with aggression. "If a boy in an unguarded moment tries to entice you to masturbatic experiments," Hall warned young audiences in a 1903 lecture presented to the American Medical Association, "he insults you. Strike him at once and beat him as long as you can stand." This reaction may sound surprising from an expert in mental health, but in fact Hall was merely following in the well-established path of such nineteenth-century medical men as Homer Bostwick and Démétrius-Alexandre Zambaco: in the face of such a dire threat, violence was all to the good.

Even the less conventional psychiatrists could not really free themselves from the centuries-old preoccupation that masturbation harmed body, mind, and soul. The revolutionary English sexologist Havelock Ellis (1859–1939), for example (whose groundbreaking *Studies in the Psychology of Sex*—first published in 1900—was, in the United States, legally available only to medical professionals until 1935), could not entirely surmount the myths. Though he endorsed "auto-erotism" and dismissed the old doctors' tales as ludicrous if not pathetic, Ellis remained nervous about "excessive masturbation," a phrase that haunted psychoanalytic writings of the era without ever being clearly defined. Ellis believed that too much solitary sex could affect the skin, the digestive system, and the circulation, and cause headache, nervous problems, and "an aversion for coitus in later life." Once again, the thought that young people might be having sex before marriage, or on their own, upset the social conventions both medicine and society felt obliged to protect and enforce.

The same was true of two of the greatest psychoanalysts of the century, Sigmund Freud (1856–1939) and his disciple Ernest Jones (1879–1958). Though these two theorists were willing to shock the world with their broad views of the sexual lives of children and adults, they still held on to anxieties about masturbation. Freud argued that the practice might lead to organic injury, permanent reductions in potency, and a "fixation of infantile sexual aims." Jones concurred. Excessive onanism, he pronounced, could lead to neurasthenia, and clitoral self-stimulation deadened sexual response. Exceptionally, one German psychoanalyst, Wilhelm Stekel (1868–1940), condemned abstinence and endorsed both masturbation and homosexuality: "Let us, once for all," Stekel urged, "abolish the fiction of normalcy in sexual matters." This position, however, was far too radical for the psychoanalytic establishment. Freud explicitly rejected Stekel's plea, which sank to the silent bottom of psychiatric seas.

If the leading intellects of the early twentieth century remained chary of masturbation, the mainstream was even more fearful. The founder of the Boy Scouts, Baron Robert Stephenson Smyth Baden-Powell (1857–1941) told his young charges that self-abuse "brings with it weakness of head and heart, and, if persisted in, idiocy and lunacy."[41] The United States government agreed. Booklets published by the U.S. Department of Labor's Children's Bureau (*Infant Care* [1914], and *Child Care* [1918]) cautioned mothers about the dangers of self-abuse in children, large, medium-sized, and small. Older children were to be warned that playing with their sex organs could stunt their growth. Babies were not exempt from risk: even in infants, the Department of Labor warned, masturbation was "an injurious practice that must be eradicated as soon as it is discovered," lest the children be "wrecked for life." Obviously, parents could not persuade babies to change their behavior; instead, they had to tie them down. "A thick towel or pad may be used to keep the thighs apart, or at night the hands may have to be restrained by pinning the nightgown sleeves to the bed, or the feet may be tied one to either side of the crib." Pacifiers—which Freud had declared autoerotic—were to be removed from the baby's mouth and "destroyed." In spite of this savagery, however, Mrs. Max West, the author of *Infant Care,* scolded parents that harsh punishments had no place in the nurturing of "a sensitive being endowed with all the desires, inclinations, and tendencies" of adults. Avoiding the dangers of masturbation, however, apparently justified whatever measures parents felt were necessary.

SEX O'CLOCK

Sexual mores began to loosen in the 1920s. Popular books like Dr. Harland Long's *Sane Sex Life and Sane Sex Living* (1919) and Dr. Lee Harlan Stone's *It Is Sex O'Clock* (1928) fiercely condemned Victorian prudery and taught acceptance of sex practices like cunnilingus and (moderate) masturbation. Even *Infant Care,* the guardian of convention, softened its tone. The 1929 edition of this little book gave parents new counsel: if they punished children for masturbation, they might only reinforce the "undesirable" behavior. Better to be psychologically savvy, the new Mrs. West advised, and distract them with a toy.

Still, some sources were more conservative. *Scouting for Girls,* the official handbook of the Girl Scouts, made quite a point in its 1920 edition about the tenth Girl Scout "law," which affirmed that "A Girl Scout Is Clean in Thought, Word, and Deed." Without actually naming such unpleasant subjects as masturbation, venereal disease, pregnancy, or sex per se, the text talked about "the deep and vital need for clean and healthy bodies in the mothers of the next generation." When questions about proper behavior arose, the handbook advised that "it is a pretty safe rule for a Girl Scout not to read things nor discuss things nor do things that could not be read nor discussed nor done by a Patrol all together." Having less fevered imaginations than Dr. Zambaco or Dr. Kellogg, the authors of *Scouting for Girls* presumably assumed that this word to the wise would be sufficient to discourage any sexual behavior, whether performed in couples, in troops, or alone.

Even as late as the 1930s and early 1940s, the rear guard continued to view masturbation as a disease. A standard pediatric textbook in 1938 still urged restraining children who played with their sexual organs. One recommended device, for example, was a rod "terminating at each end with a leather collar," used to keep the child's knees apart while he or she slept. Circumcision of penis and clitoris were approved operations. The U.S. Naval Academy at Annapolis in 1940 still officially rejected candidates who displayed "evidence of masturbation," and the 1942 *Infant Care* still classed masturbation as an undesirable habit, in the evil company of "Thumb Sucking" and "Playing with Stool." In 1945, the *Boy Scout Manual* continued to warn against self-abuse, and psychoanalyst Otto Fenichel wrote that masturbation was "clearly pathological" when patients preferred it to intercourse.[42]

Old attitudes had clearly not died out by the late 1940s, when Dr. Benjamin Spock published his *Common Sense Book of Baby and Child Care.* Spock felt obliged to caution his readers that it was wise to avoid circumcision "after the baby is a few months old, certainly as a treatment for masturbation." He also recorded the story of two parents who "were morbidly afraid of masturbation. They hired a companion for their [adolescent] son whose job it was to stay close to him 24 hours a day, to make sure he didn't do it." The result of this monitoring, Spock observed, was to make the boy both obsessed with masturbation and terrified of its consequences. Attitudes were changing, but they had clearly not all changed yet.

Even when the medical establishment backed away from these stances in the 1940s and 1950s, masturbation remained freighted with guilt. Marie Stopes (1880–1958), the author of a popular sex manual called *Married Love,* received thousands of letters about sex from troubled Americans from the end of World War I until World War II. As historian Lesley L. Hall notes, correspondents of the later generation were no less fearful about masturbation than their parents had been.[43]

One uprising against the history of guilt and shame came from sex surveys, which disclosed the fact that large majorities of the European and American populaces masturbated. If 90 to 100 percent of men had engaged in the practice, as a Berlin study showed in 1895, how could the habit be dangerous or wrong? These figures were bolstered by later data. A 1929 study by Katherine Bement Davis, a University of Chicago Ph.D. who advised John D. Rockefeller, Jr.'s, Bureau of Social Hygiene, found that 64.8 percent of unmarried women and 40.1 percent of married women acknowledged the practice—a figure likely to be only a portion of those who actually carried it out.[44]

These figures were corroborated by the famous Indiana University sexologist Alfred Kinsey (1894–1956). Studying American sex habits with the passion for detail that had hallmarked his training as an entomologist, Kinsey bowled the country over with his revelations. Almost as startling as his widely quoted statistic that 10 percent of American men had had homosexual experiences, his views on masturbation raised eyebrows and ire. Kinsey asserted that masturbation was normal and even beneficial; he thundered against repressive attitudes, criticized Freud, and argued that women who masturbated before marriage felt more wedded bliss than their chaster peers.

Kinsey's attitudes opened eyes, but they did not win him lasting favor. In the early 1950s, investigated by Congress and condemned by religious groups, he lost the major funding for his Institute for Sex Research; under this pressure, his health collapsed. The attitudes Kinsey had protested were still strong enough to wreck his career and shorten his life.

This slow and hesitant evolution was evident on the theological side as well. A book entitled *New Views on Sex-Marriage-Love*, written by Frederick von Gagern, M.D., and published in 1968 with the imprimatur of the Roman Catholic Church, saw masturbation as the sign of "an unresolved problem in the individual's life." Still using eighteenth-century terminology, this physician observed that what the "onanist" needed was not condemnation or moral advice, but "help." In 1970, the forward-looking Catholic University theologian Charles E. Curran took a milder point of view in his book *Contemporary Problems in Moral Theology*. Curran argued that masturbation was not always a "grave matter," and urged that it not prevent adolescents from receiving holy communion. Curran's radical views on sex, however, led the Vatican to tell him in 1986 that he would "no longer be considered suitable nor eligible to exercise the function of professor of Catholic theology."[45]

Even in the 1990s, masturbation is still a dirty word. Forty years after Kinsey and a century after Kellogg, a 1995 textbook of psychiatry noted that approximately 50 percent of American men and women felt guilty for masturbating. When Dr. Joycelyn Elders remarked that masturbation "is part of human sexuality," and suggested it be taught as a way of preventing AIDS, President Bill Clinton removed her from her position as his surgeon general. And 1996 materials from the Medical Institute for Sexual Health, a conservative Texas foundation dedicated to reducing pregnancy and sexually transmitted disease among teenagers, frowned on the idea that masturbation should receive positive mention in high-school sex education curricula. Though masturbation is no longer automatically linked with disease, it retains its role as a sex practice that no one can separate from its layers of guilt and social taboo.

AN ALL-PURPOSE CULPRIT

It is clear that, for three hundred years, the medical profession and the public alike believed that masturbation made people morally, physically, and mentally sick. But *why* did they believe this? And how do these attitudes, like the others I discuss in this book, relate to broader issues of sex and health?

The first question to answer is whether there was some real, historical change around 1700 that provoked the medical profession to react so strongly. Historians suggest that, in fact, people may well have begun to masturbate more in the eighteenth century than they had done in the decades and centuries before: as Enlightenment historian Théodore Tarczylo has noted, the new concern about masturbation may well have indicated a changing social reality. If so, the new behavior could have increased both awareness and anxiety, especially in an area already as troubled as sex.

French historian Michelle Perrot notes that people's private lives changed significantly at this time. Europeans were marrying later, she explains, and the social attitudes that had once winked at limited premarital sex grew more intrusive and more rigid; this meant that young people had fewer sexual outlets. In addition, the young spent more time alone. Whereas before they had been constantly in the midst of their families, now they had beds and bedrooms of their own. They attended single-sex schools; young men found living quarters in "veritable bachelors' ghettoes" in the cities. Furthermore, increasing rates of syphilis and gonorrhea may have made sexual intercourse less appealing. Some young people no doubt chose celibacy; others, however, probably had sex less often with partners and more often by themselves.

It is also true that some of the fears doctors cited were in fact confirmed by Kinsey's data. Boys, the Indiana researcher found, typically learned how to masturbate from other boys, while girls more often made the discovery on their own. Three percent of girls and nine percent of boys learned to masturbate from homosexual experience, a recurrent medical and social fear. Worst of all, tasting the apple from the Tree of Knowledge of Good and Evil did indeed lead to sin: once people found that they *could* masturbate, most immediately *did.* The stories were true, though their dangers were imaginary.

So it seems likely that, at least from 1700 on, many (or even most) Europeans and Americans masturbated. But why did they think it made them sick? This question has many answers. Some came from the history of the medical profession. The antique doctrine of the humors held sway until the eighteenth century, and even later than this physicians believed that expending semen had to damage the body's health. (Social morality, however, conveniently helped people forget that classical medicine had warned that abstinence was as dangerous as sexual overindulgence.) Masturbation was also an easy scapegoat for medical problems doctors could not solve. Since so many people (and, especially, so many young people) practiced it, doctors could argue that there was a connection between masturbation and almost any illness. This correlation was particularly valuable in an era when physicians could diagnose far more diseases than they could actually cure: as historian Arthur Gilbert points out, children's masturbation "became an all-purpose culprit for a medical profession that could not provide answers for grieving parents." If children died from tuberculosis (a major killer not fully understood until the 1890s), if patients suffered from gout, asthma, eating disorders, rickets, heart disease, or hemorrhoids, the cause could always be diagnosed as self-abuse. Since so many people did masturbate, and since they believed that what they were doing to their bodies was making them sick, patients were readily persuaded to believe their doctors and blame themselves.

AN UNTIMELY AND FEARFUL END

This pattern showed through in a haunting story recounted by New York surgeon Homer Bostwick: the case of "Miss R., aged seventeen, the daughter of a highly respectable merchant of this city." Bostwick was called to the R. family's house on 10 May 1846, and was deeply shocked by the stark contrast between the home's external prosperity and the shameful and sorrowful events transpiring within its walls.

On arriving, the surgeon found his young patient propped up in bed, her face displaying a "calm smile of resignation." She knew that death held her firmly within its grasp. Once her parents had left the room, the girl confessed everything to her doctor. She attributed her rapid consumption to the habit of onanism, which had taken hold of her at an early age. Knowing its dangers did nothing to stop her, and though she was sorry at her ruin, she was hardly surprised. All she hoped for was that, once she was gone, the doctor would advise her mother to discover and correct in her two younger sisters "what she never seemed to observe in me, and thus save her children from so untimely and fearful an end as mine. This, doctor, is my last request." Destroyed by her own hand, as Bostwick judged, the girl died a few days later, leaving behind only a grieving family and a cautionary tale.

The tuberculosis this girl diagnosed may well have carried her off. Many other patients who thought they were suffering from the harmful effects of masturbation probably suffered from gonorrhea, a disease that has been around since the beginnings of human history. With its symptomatic discharges, urinary blockage, female sterility, and blinding eye infections, gonorrhea corresponds closely to many of the symptoms eighteenth- and nineteenth-century doctors ascribed to onanism.

This hypothesis is borne out by the high rates of gonorrhea nineteenth-century doctors reported. Steinhardt warned boys that 70 to 80 percent of all men who had sex with prostitutes became infected; Hall asserted that 60 to 75 percent of all men had had gonorrhea by the age of thirty. High as these figures are, they may not have been entirely off base. A man infected with gonorrhea passes the disease to half of his sexual partners, a woman to one partner in five. From the 1950s to the 1980s, 1 to 2 percent of Americans had active cases of gonorrhea at any given time, even though the disease does not linger and effective treatment was readily available. In Africa, where treatment is harder to find, rates are much higher—three to ten per hundred. Rates in the United States and Europe before the age of antibiotics could easily have been comparable: even today, sexually transmitted diseases are the most common infections in America.

Even more alarming is a fact reported by Richard Rothenberg of the Centers for Disease Control. Most children with gonorrhea today, Rothenberg states, have acquired it through sexual abuse. What transpired in the infected shadows of the Victorian era? Some children may have chosen to blame their symptoms on masturbation, rather than report even more dreadful crimes.

Eighteenth- and nineteenth-century fears of childhood sexuality, both hetero- and homo-, may also have betrayed the seductive and dangerous appeal of adolescents to adults. Why did Dr. Kellogg dwell so longingly on the "crimson petals tightly folded" beneath the "swelling bud" of adolescent girls? What moved Dr. Winfield Hall to linger over the hard and growing bodies of teenaged boys, the "masculine shoulders, massive hips, and swelling muscles" of those fully grown? The young of this era were not the only ones with sexual secrets to hide.

In the case of the mentally ill, physicians are likely to have mistaken symptom for cause. In the eighteenth and nineteenth centuries, more and more people with mental handicaps were confined to asylums. Whatever these patients had done in private in their bedrooms was now on public display in the hospital wards. Mental illness often removes inhibitions; frequent and public masturbation may well have been a symptom of other problems. Some of the incarcerated, of course, had been designated as crazy simply *because* they masturbated—hardly surprising in an age when mental illness was attributed to a wide range of human troubles. As the archives of the Pennsylvania Hospital show, "supposed causes of insanity" in the nineteenth century included "Disappointed Affections," "Intense Study," "Metaphysical Speculations," "Exposure to Direct Rays of the Sun," "Religious Excitement," "Celibacy," "Mortified Pride," "Use of Tobacco," "Childbirth," "Tight Lacing," "Political Excitement," "Nostalgia," "Want of Exercise," "Sudden Acquisition of Wealth," "Menopause," and "Stock Speculations." Masturbation was hardly more far-fetched a cause of insanity than these.

Other patients were suffering from problems we would now call by different names. The patient Tissot described as "a being that less resembled a living creature than a corpse" was probably afflicted with advanced neurosyphilis. The "obstinacy, sadness, . . . indifference . . . and melancholy" Wilhelm Gollmann described are symptoms of clinical depression. The two little Turkish girls tortured by Dr. Zambaco's cautery irons may have been brain-damaged, or they may have been acting out in response to parental sexual abuse. The four-year-old girl in Berlin who "passed hour after hour in a corner, her tongue lolling from her mouth" would now be described as autistic; her miraculous cure by clitoridectomy would be considered medical propaganda. Like mental illness, these problems were real, but masturbation was at most their symptom, not their cause.[46] French concerns about underpopulation, Victorian English fears of female sexuality, and the Puritanical democracy of the United States all played a role as well.[47]

True, sexual morality in the eighteenth and nineteenth centuries became less and less religious and more and more medical, but the morality itself was essentially unchanged. If anything, the halo of learning and science that adorned the medical profession reinforced existing structures of social control. Masturbation was a way for people to escape from these bonds; that is why it was dangerous. Physicians knew this; the public knew it, too. All were equally frightened.

Precisely because it is so different from current ideas of disease, masturbation—like lovesickness—provides a screen on which we can clearly view the sexual morality and beliefs of an earlier era. What the study of masturbation shows is that for two and a half centuries people quickly panicked over sexual behavior that fell outside the approved norms. Guided by authority, they garbed their fears in medical clothing. They agreed that, with God and nature as moral enforcers, solitary sexual behavior would lead to disease and death, and that it was up to the medical profession to rescue masturbators from themselves. All too happily, the medical profession—populated by such figures as Drs. Tissot, Bostwick, Zambaco, and Kellogg—readily concurred. The damage they did to their patients, and which their patients did to themselves, survives in masturbation's legacy of anxiety and fear.

CHAPTER SIX

AIDS in the U.S.A.

Far more recent and familiar than any period I have so far touched upon, and yet in some ways distant almost beyond recall, the 1960s and 1970s were the halcyon days of modern medicine. During this brief *pax antibiotica*, as one writer has called it, the heavy gates of the Temple of Disease appeared finally to have swung shut with a resounding clang. Penicillin and a host of new drugs seemed to be making infectious disease a thing of the past; vaccines were developed to prevent many of the crueler afflictions of childhood, such as polio, typhoid, and diphtheria. In an extraordinarily ambitious and effective worldwide campaign, smallpox was eradicated. Looking at a future in which the only major health problems would be chronic ones like cancer and heart disease, universities began to shut down their departments of infectious disease and tropical medicine, while some cities withdrew funds from the public clinics they had long provided to control such afflictions as tuberculosis.

Particularly in Europe and the United States, these transformations were felt on the sexual front as well. Old scourges like syphilis and gonorrhea were now seen as minor nuisances that could be cured with a couple of shots; concerns about masturbation had more or less faded from view; and prophylactics, contraceptives, and abortion were increasingly socially accepted and easy to obtain. Coupled with these factors was a series of social movements that drastically changed people's concepts of the meaning and place of sex in their lives: the sexual revolution, feminism, and the beginnings of the modern gay and lesbian movement. Suddenly, much of the population felt much freer to be sexually active than it had in decades, and the accidental consequences of sex—pregnancy and infection—seemed more remote than they had ever been. Sex outside of wedlock was safe; it was readily available; it was viewed as liberating; and—perhaps most important of all, in the consumer culture of the United States—sex was fun.

Into this petri dish of social change dropped the virus that would come to be known as HIV. This microscopic particle would reveal the flaws in many of the assumptions that had governed recent views of sex, disease, and many other parts of life. The freedom and openness with which men and women viewed casual sex, the safety with which many viewed heterosexual marriage, the strength of national borders and the belief that science could control the threats of the natural world—all of these comfortable assumptions were challenged and weakened by the power of a diminutive parasite that was not really even alive.

This chapter will look at the history of some of these troubles and challenges in the United States in the years since 1981. My focus here will be the same as it was in earlier chapters—the way in which society linked this disease to traditional views of sex and sin. Some parts of the story were painfully familiar; many old notions, like that of "innocent victims," and of disease as a divine punishment for sin, enjoyed a renaissance that would have seemed unthinkable in previous years. Other parts of the story were new. One of these was a sense of group identity among the afflicted. There is not much evidence that people suffering from leprosy, syphilis, or medical treatment for masturbation thought of themselves as a class, a group of people defined by their illness and entitled to rights because of it. With AIDS, however—especially in the early years, when the disease was closely identified with the emerging minority of gay men—people with AIDS took on a collective voice, and fought back against the social forces they saw as oppressing them. Another was the government. Unlike the battles over earlier diseases, which primarily took place in doctors' offices, learned journals, and confessionals, America's loud and belligerent disagreements about AIDS took place on the far more public terrain of the White House, the Congress, federal agencies, and courtrooms, as well as the local fronts of subways, schools, and city halls. There was a tremendous amount of name-calling; there were accusations and counteraccusations; there were lawsuits and lies. More important, there were deaths in enormous numbers. The devastation caused by AIDS paralleled that of many of

history's gravest epidemics, and, like these earlier scourges, AIDS ultimately hit hardest those who were least able to take care of themselves.

The history of AIDS pulls together many of the major themes of this
book. Like lepers, some people with AIDS have been stigmatized and
excluded from society; like syphilitics and those stricken with plague,
some have been blamed for being sick and accused of bringing catastrophe down not only on their own heads, but also on the heads of the
so-called innocent. As with masturbation and lovesickness, the debate
about AIDS focused regularly on prevention and the question of
whether certain kinds of sexual activity were benign or harmful in
themselves—and whether they could be discussed in public. Despite
the profound differences between late twentieth-century America and
the periods discussed in previous chapters, the guilt, the accusations,
and the patterns of blame hearkened back through time, recalling moralists and moralities one might have imagined—*I* had imagined—were
dead and gone. These turned out to be not only alive but widespread
and powerful: the past was present again. Like Francis Herring, the
seventeenth-century English author who described plague as "the
stroke of God's wrath for the sins of mankind," the Reverend Jerry Falwell felt free to proclaim to a national television audience in 1987 that
"a God who hates sin has stopped [homosexuality] dead in its tracks by
saying, 'do it and die.' 'Do it and die.'"[1]

These views surfaced with extraordinary frequency in the 1980s, both
across the nation and on Capitol Hill. The belief that AIDS was a punishment God had visited on a perverse group of sinners not only colored
the national discourse and made many of those who were sick or afraid
feel even more guilty and anxious than they already were; it also took
on legal force and had drastic consequences for the health of the nation.
Because some people believed that AIDS was a punishment for immoral behavior, federal and state agencies were forbidden to give complete and accurate information about prevention to the public. Because
some institutions believed that condoms were not to be mentioned in
public or in the schools, municipalities failed to teach their teenagers
what they needed to know to avoid infection. The avoidable consequence, in every case, was that many people continued to have unprotected sex and share infected needles, become HIV-positive, fall sick,
and die.

It would be foolish and inaccurate to assert that better prevention
programs alone would have stopped the American AIDS epidemic
short. It is tremendously difficult to change human sexual behavior, and

people often will ignore the best advice, even when their own lives are at risk. But, at least in the United States, things could have been different, could have been better, could have been less severe. The following pages tell tales of misguided priorities, of missed opportunities, and also of some exemplary cases in which things turned out for the best—cases that may serve as better models for the future.

Right Living

As it began to spread around the country in the late 1970s and early 1980s, HIV found America a complex and divided nation, particularly in regard to sex. At one extreme was the political and religious right, which publicly espoused—and sometimes tried to enforce—old and often highly romanticized patterns of sex and gender behavior: compulsory heterosexuality, virginity until marriage and strict monogamy afterward, and gender roles in which wives were subservient to husbands. To these ideals, traditional Catholics added an abhorrence of condoms and contraception and a complete ban on abortions; some Protestants were also exceptionally troubled by and opposed to homosexuality. As Scott Appleby, associate director of the American Academy of Arts and Sciences' Fundamentalism Project, put it, to religious conservatives "the AIDS epidemic, pornography, a rising divorce rate, teen-aged pregnancy, and, especially, abortion are read not simply as society's failings, but as clear warnings of something much worse at work, the forces of evil struggling with God for mastery of this planet."[2]

Making anal sex safer for homosexuals was nowhere on the agenda of the religious right, which saw it as natural and proper that activities like this had dangerous consequences that it would be reckless and even immoral to minimize. In many ways, conservatives believed, America was on the wrong track, and AIDS was a critical warning sign. The only real way to stop the threat to America's health, as Sen. Jesse Helms explained, was to "slam the door on the wayward, wanton sexual revolution which has ravaged this Nation."[3] In a perfect world, as imagined by the religious right, sexually transmitted diseases would vanish in a generation because all promiscuity would come to a halt—a vision resembling that of the second- and third-century Christians who endorsed universal celibacy, hoping that through this means the kingdom of God would soon come to hand.

Homosexuality was perhaps the flashiest of all the failings conservatives saw in modern life, and it was hardly surprising that the conspicuous and vocal emergence of a national gay rights movement in the 1970s should have caught and held the attention of the religious right as it did. In the eyes of many Christians, notes a leading expert on fundamentalism, the University of Chicago Divinity School's Martin Marty, "to engage in sex with a member of one's own gender is not just immoral, or a lamentable but understandable weakness, but a perversion of nature, an abomination in the sight of God, an act deserving of imprisonment and perhaps even death."[4] With these views layered on top of the history of sex and disease outlined in the preceding chapters, it was hardly surprising that AIDS should have fallen like a spark in a powder keg. Many of the religious and political right rose to the task of reading God's message in the new disease and denouncing the homosexuals they believed had inflicted it on an overly tolerant nation. Falwell, for example, claimed in the spring of 1987 that

> AIDS is a lethal judgment of God on the sin of homosexuality and it is also the judgment of God on America for endorsing this vulgar, perverted, and reprobate lifestyle. . . . God destroyed Sodom and Gomorrah primarily because of the sin of homosexuality. Today, He is again bringing judgment against this wicked practice through AIDS.[5]

For Reverend Falwell and those agreed with his principles, homosexuality was America's most flagrant failing, and AIDS God's righteous response.

Many conservatives were as eager to blame homosexuals for the AIDS epidemic as their forefathers had been to assert that syphilis was the fault of sailors, Neapolitans, prostitutes, or the French. AIDS was "nature's form of retribution," political columnist and perennial presidential candidate Pat Buchanan explained, for the "immoral, unnatural, unsanitary, unhealthy, and suicidal practice of anal intercourse." Jerry Falwell's *Moral Majority Report* put the same sentiment into a punchier phrase: "What gays do to each other," it noted, "makes them sick and, more and more frequently, dead!" The note these commentators sounded was partly a warning bell, and partly a peal of jubilation at seeing their views confirmed: the wicked truly *were* punished in this life. But beneath the approbation was a heavy undertone of fear. The *Moral Majority Report* warned that AIDS was turning up in "exponentially increasing numbers of defenseless heterosexuals" who happened to cross the sinners' deadly path. Buchanan saw AIDS emanating from the perverted and tainted bodies of the nation's homosexuals and drug users like the ripples in a pond. The virus, he wrote, spread from the guilty to the innocent, from the dirty city streets to the sacred suburban home, from "the needles of IV drug users, the transfusions of hemophiliacs, and the bloodstreams of unsuspecting health workers [and] prostitutes [to] lovers, wives, children."[6] By 1987, Jesse Helms could reduce the idea to a simple, if inaccurate, principle: "Every AIDS case can be traced back to a homosexual act."[7]

Throughout the first decade of the epidemic, these views combined with Americans' fears to create an atmosphere hostile to people with AIDS. In 1983, physicians at the National Institutes of Health grumbled that gay men had brought the new disease upon themselves, and *Science* magazine fulminated about the "unprecedented spending spree" lavished on AIDS research—a perception radically at odds with the fiscal realities.[8] President Reagan's budget proposal for fiscal 1984, for example, reduced real spending for the CDC by 7 percent, and the NIH, in the same year, allocated to AIDS only $9.4 million—.002 of its budget.[9]

Surveys found similar views among the public. A 1988 study published in the *Journal of the American Medical Association* found that 60 percent of those polled felt "not much" or "no" sympathy for people who had been infected with HIV through homosexual sex; almost 30 percent wanted to quarantine those infected. Between 20 and 25 percent of Americans (and 33 percent of Southerners) explicitly favored discriminating against people with AIDS; one in five said AIDS patients were "offenders who were getting their rightful due."[10] Four years later, 27 percent still felt that people with AIDS should *not* be treated with compassion.[11] Conservative politicians were quick to confirm the belief that AIDS was a punishment for sin. AIDS, explained William Bennett, President Reagan's secretary of education, showed how "harsh nature becomes the unwitting ally of responsible morality." Archconservative California congressman Robert ("B-1 Bob") Dornan saw AIDS as "the reaper's scythe" that cut homosexuals down in their prime.[12] HIV had not only given rise to a new disease: it had given new life to old prejudices.

With these attitudes in Washington, it was no surprise that effective prevention programs made slow progress around the nation. From the White House emanated only a ghostly silence: during the first six years of the AIDS crisis—as 59,572 Americans were diagnosed and 27,909 of them died—President Reagan never once mentioned the disease in public, as if those people, their communities, families, and friends did not exist at all. Meanwhile, his administration cut funding for all the agencies whose job it was to respond to public health problems, making exceptions only for those diseases that affected groups deemed socially acceptable: toxic shock syndrome (women), the Tylenol scare (drug-store shoppers), and Legionnaires' Disease (veterans).

ACT UP! Stop AIDS!

Strikingly different views of these topics were held by those on the other side of the HIV divide. The gay movement was far smaller, less powerful, and less well connected politically than the Christian right, but it did have one tremendous strength: for gay men, AIDS was an absolute threat not just to their habits and beliefs, but to life itself, and hence a challenge that had to be met with every possible resource. Though HIV probably began to penetrate the drug-injecting communities of the American urban poor around the same time it hit the gay community, it was the newly emergent class of middle-class gay white men who became most closely identified with and defined by the new disease. These men had a common identity, a social infrastructure that could be pulled into action, access to medical care, and a new sense of entitlement that gave them self-awareness and the willingness to speak out about their sufferings and to push for change.

In the 1960s and 1970s, the gay and lesbian movement had pursued many goals—the right to be open about sexual orientation and the right to be equal in the eyes of religious bodies and the law. But one of its earliest and most basic objectives, especially for gay men, was sexual freedom: the right to have sexual lives that were untrammeled by the conventions and limitations of society's norms. For some men, this meant monogamous, long-lasting partnerships with other men; for others, it meant looser and more complex domestic and emotional arrangements. And for many, it meant the freedom to enjoy sexual relations with many partners, either on a continuing basis or just in passing. Gay men—and many other men who outwardly lived heterosexual lives—found sex through social networks and in the many propitious settings of urban America, such as public parks, cruising areas, and the baths.

This freedom combined with three other new factors to contribute enormously to the rapid and global spread of HIV. One was the increasing ease and availability of air travel. Emerging diseases that, in the past, might have remained in isolated communities now had frequent-flyer tickets to the most populous regions of the world. Another relative novelty was the increasing flexibility of sex roles. Homosexuality in more traditional cultures had typically followed rigid patterns: certain men were the insertive partners in oral or anal intercourse, others the receptive ones. In the 1970s and 1980s, however, American gay men often took both insertive *and* receptive roles. Rather than serve as a cul-de-sac for the virus, as heterosexual women often did, gay and bisexual men more often acted as an extremely effective conduit for HIV. The virus also had another great advantage over most infections: the extended incubation period—often ten years or more—between infection and the onset of visible symptoms. People could be infected and infect many others long before anyone knew they were sick.

Despite this time lag, AIDS awareness came surprisingly early to some, including some members of the gay community.[13] In 1981, activist Larry Kramer founded an organization in New York known as the Gay Men's Health Crisis, now the nation's largest AIDS organization, and, later, a more radical group called ACT-UP (the AIDS Coalition To Unleash Power). Though Kramer himself continually reproached his peers for being promiscuous, these groups sought ways to join the gay movement's long-established goals of sexual freedom to the new one of finding a way to preserve gay men's health. Bit by bit, they adopted a program known as "safe" (and then, more realistically, "safer") sex. Its principles were simple: that what was dangerous was not homosexual sex per se, but sex that involved the transmission of infected fluids—semen, vaginal fluid, breast milk, blood. The proponents of safer sex looked for ways to eroticize condoms and nonpenetrative sex, to inform people about the dangers of HIV, and to persuade them to practice and enjoy activities that would keep them virus-free.

Scientific evidence quickly piled up in support of the principles of safer sex. Condoms, for example, proved highly effective in stopping the spread of HIV. One European study showed that condoms prevented viral transmission in mixed-status couples who used them consistently; studies in Thailand, Uganda, Ethiopia, and Kenya showed that condoms prevented HIV transmission even in the challenging conditions of the developing world.[14] A condom campaign in Switzerland in the late 1980s brought the level of unprotected sex among young people down from 81 percent to 27 percent.[15] American data were consistent with these results. When Surgeon General C. Everett Koop endorsed condom use in 1986, sales doubled.[16] A study published in *JAMA* in 1991 showed that even hard-to-reach populations, such as runaway youth in shelters, doubled their rate of condom use and dramatically cut down on unsafe sexual activity after intensive counseling and education.[17] And in San Francisco, after major national campaigns, the rate of HIV infection among gay men dropped from 6,000–8,000 per year in the early 1980s to only 1,000 in 1992.[18] These promising statistics were reinforced by the startling epidemiological fact that if Americans' risky behavior were reduced by half, the AIDS epidemic would simply fade away.[19] Safer sex, if widely observed, protected both the individuals who practiced it and the health of the nation.

These studies and statistics persuaded the leaders of the gay anti-AIDS movement, who were gradually joined by most of the American public health establishment. Battles for public support and programs, however, remained. Safer gay and extramarital sex was obviously not a goal that conservative and religious groups would endorse, and in the 1980s political map of the American skies, Republican constellations shone much brighter than those of GMHC or ACT-UP. The radical right and the activist left fought over two related prizes: the faith and trust of the American people, and the policies of the American government. Much of the epidemic's future would hinge on how these battles went.

Gradually, AIDS prevention policies did emerge, some good, some bad. The overall trends in America were positive: eventually, repressive rules were lifted, accurate prevention messages were disseminated, and prejudices, to a large degree, were replaced by sympathy. The struggles leading up to each of these developments, however, were great. Progress was slow and costly; thousands died needlessly. Prevention—even today the most important weapon against AIDS by far—continues to be misunderstood, underfunded, and ineffectual; prejudices remain. These events unfolded in all parts of government (the White House, Congress, and the courts), as well as in cities and states throughout the country.

THE SURGEON GENERAL REPORTS ON AIDS

"It was not easy for a grandfather of seventy years, been married for fifty, to be out talking about condoms on television and radio," admitted C. Everett Koop in a 1997 interview. Certainly, if anyone had to pick the national figure of the 1980s most likely to be discussing condoms on TV, it would not have been Dr. Koop. Bearded, bespectacled, outspokenly Christian, professional, and gruff, Koop nearly failed to be confirmed as surgeon general because much of America considered him to be too conservative for the post. In retrospect, however, he was one of the most influential proponents of AIDS prevention in the Reagan and Bush years. How did this happen?

Koop's background would not have led people to suspect that he would take such a view. He had come to Reagan's attention through the offices of the Reverend Billy Graham, who had heard of Koop as a vehement opponent of abortion—as indeed he was. An Evangelical Christian, Koop and another author had written a book and made a documentary film about abortion in 1977, both provocatively titled *Whatever Happened to the Human Race?* As historian William C. Martin recounts,

> *Whatever Happened to the Human Race?* was not a subtle production. In one arresting scene from the film, Koop stands in shallow water near the shoreline of the Dead Sea, which he identifies as the site of the former city of Sodom. As Koop intones, "Sodom comes easily to mind when one contemplates the evils of abortion and the death of moral law," one notices that all about him in every direction are hundreds of dolls, representing the one million babies aborted each year in the wake of the *Roe vs. Wade* decision. No one had to wonder where Everett Koop stood on the question of abortion.[20]

This was precisely the kind of person the Reagan administration wanted in charge of the Public Health Service. Koop's stand on abortion, however, was not as popular with the rest of the country as it was with the Reagan crowd. Enthusiastic backing from the right was nearly outmatched by the ferocious opposition of the country's liberal establishment, which assaulted the nomination en bloc. A remarkable array of forces, including the American Medical Association, the American Public Health Association, Planned Parenthood, the National Gay Health Coalition, and thirteen major dailies opposed Koop; the *New York Times* denounced him as "Dr. Unqualified." Despite the attacks, however, the Senate confirmed Koop's appointment to the post of surgeon general.

What Koop's conservative backers had not really understood, however, was that even though the Philadelphia surgeon was a serious Christian, his values on other issues did not line up squarely with theirs. Koop's antiabortion stand grew out of his religious belief that life and health were sacred; these were the same convictions that motivated his medical work. Koop followed a party line quite strictly, but it was his own party line, and there was more than one place where it ran perpendicular to that of the people who had put him in power.

One area of conflict was smoking. Early in his tenure, Koop challenged Republican support for cigarette advertising, siding with liberal Democratic congressman Henry Waxman (a former opponent) against the Reagan White House, the Department of Justice, and Senator Helms. Another was AIDS. The new disease was a natural topic of concern for the surgeon general, as it had been for Koop since early on; the administration, however, made it clear that, on this matter, the surgeon general was to maintain a monastic silence. On AIDS as on tobacco advertising, the Reagan administration put politics before the national health. These politics were explained in a 1997 interview by Gary Bauer, a protégé of Secretary of Education William Bennett who became head of the White House's main political office, the Domestic Policy Council. The council's job was to determine which American issues the administration handled, and how. "Any White House," Bauer told me, "tries to dissociate itself or not to be too closely connected with, a 'bad news' story," and AIDS was as bad as they come. Homosexuality, intravenous drugs, incurable disease, and death—these were hardly the kind of topics with which Bauer and his colleagues wanted the president and his people to be connected. Furthermore, Bauer's knowledge and objectivity were questioned by the member of his staff responsible for AIDS issues. "To my knowledge, [Bauer] never really knew what was going on. He didn't understand AIDS at all. All he knew was what was going on with some evangelical groups, and things that were causing them discomfort he would kill and things they liked he would push and that was the total extent of his interest in AIDS."[21]

The result of these views was a gag order on the surgeon general. AIDS activists and the news media kept raising the issue; Koop himself was anxious to speak out. But for five and a half years, the surgeon general was forbidden by his direct superior, the assistant secretary for health, even to mention the epidemic in public. "Whenever I spoke on a health issue at a press conference or on a network morning TV show," Koop recalled, "the government public affairs people told the media in advance that I would not answer questions on AIDS, and I was not to be asked any questions on the subject"—the subject that was becoming the defining public health issue of the decade.

Only around 1986 did the veil of silence begin to lift. Perhaps because his friend Rock Hudson had at last acknowledged that he had AIDS, Reagan finally began to address the issue, albeit with little enthusiasm. "Quite casually," Koop recalled, the president asked him in 1986 to prepare a report to the American people on the epidemic. (The president did not mention AIDS in public until a 1987 visit to the College of Physicians of Philadelphia, where he announced that the only prevention policy the nation needed was to "just say no.") Koop took his assignment far more seriously than the president's tone might have indicated, gathering all the information he could obtain—especially on prevention. And because he was aware of the delicate politics involved,

Koop also spent weeks and weeks canvassing every pertinent special interest group he could think of, from the United States Catholic Conference to the National Coalition of Black Lesbians and Gays. His goal was to produce a report that was accurate and informative, but that would not offend the American public.

The surgeon general succeeded on one of these two counts: the report he released on 22 October 1986, with the approval of the new HHS secretary, Otis Bowen, was clinical and accurate. It was also remarkably frank. It endorsed abstinence, but was not shy about explaining that AIDS could be transmitted by anal, oral, or vaginal sex—and that transmission could be prevented by the proper use of condoms.

The report was sent to health professionals, but Koop had a far larger public in mind: he wanted to do what the British government had done, and send an information sheet about AIDS to every household in the nation. At this, the political forces in the Reagan administration became truly alarmed. To many people, both the topic and the recommendations of the report were scandalous and even immoral. The thought that a member of a conservative administration would send to every household in America a mailer discussing topics like anal sex and warning people to confront their spouses about infidelity ("It's your life," the brochure reminded its readers) would be politically disastrous.

Reflecting back on those days, Bauer talked about the administration's fiscal and epidemiological concerns. To send information about AIDS to every household in the country would be silly, he argued.

> There was already adequate evidence at the time to know that the at-risk population was not a seventy-year-old woman in Iowa. But it was, in fact, by and large, young gay men, IV drug users—and, even then, increasingly, minority members. And so we argued for a long time over the use of scarce federal dollars, and argued that the mailing, particularly if it was going to be explicit, ought to be targeted to the target population. And for that, we were constantly accused of trying to censor material.

This argument was partly accurate: elderly women in Iowa were not particularly likely to be exposed to HIV, as the report made clear. But wasting a sheet of newsprint and a stamp was not the crucial issue here. Much more troubling—particularly to conservative Christians—was that the administration might be discussing sex in an "explicit" manner. If the cost of avoiding this problem meant that "young gay men, IV drug users, and minority members" (none of them strong Republican constituencies) did not get full and clear prevention information, that was a cost the administration might be willing to bear. In the eyes of

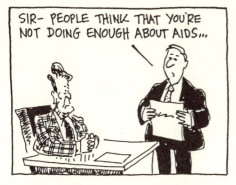
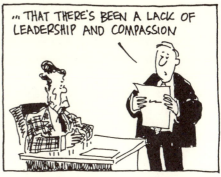
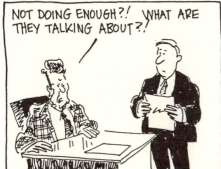
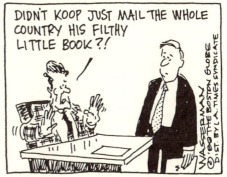

"The Surgeon General's Report on AIDS." Dan Wasserman cartoon. © 1988, *Boston Globe*. Distributed by Los Angeles Times Syndicate. Reprinted by permission.

some members of the administration, people like this simply did not exist. Koop recalled that, at a White House Domestic Policy Council meeting on the topic, one staffer "objected to the statement in the AIDS report that 'most Americans are opposed to homosexuality, promiscuity of any kind, and prostitution.' He wanted me to say 'All Americans . . .' and did not seem to understand that I could not say it because it was not true."[22]

The council's political calculations left these people—homosexuals, drug users, nonwhites—out in the cold; so did the fiscal calculations of the Reagan budget. Federal dollars were "scarce," as Bauer put it, not by accident but because the administration had drastically reduced money for domestic priorities by cutting taxes, inflating the military budget, and letting the federal deficit balloon to unprecedented levels—as much as $200 billion a year.

Over the administration's opposition, Congress did eventually find the funds Koop sought, and the brochure went out to 107 million households, as well as to physicians, nurses, state health departments, the military, as well as to Americans living abroad, in homeless shelters, and in prisons.[23] Once published, it met with a barrage of attacks and objections, some from the White House itself. A mere three weeks after the report was complete, for example, Bauer suggested to Koop that it be "updated" by deleting all references to condoms—an idea Koop dismissed as "ridiculous."[24] Taking another tack, Bauer's political mentor Bill Bennett decided to publish an AIDS primer of his own as an alternative to the surgeon general's brochure. Bennett admitted that parents needed to know "the facts, the often unwelcome facts" about AIDS, but in reality they were unlikely to learn many of these from his book. He recommended one resource to his readers, for example, as suitable for use because it "avoids explicit and detailed discussion of risky sexual practices and does not address the use of condoms."[25] Ignorance, to the United States secretary of education, was bliss.

On the nation's conservative exchanges, the surgeon general's stock plummeted. An organization called Concerned Women for America denounced the report as pornographic;[26] Senator Helms's staff broke off all communication with Koop. The *National Review* asserted that condoms were *not* effective at preventing viral transmission, and declared the surgeon general guilty of "criminal negligence" for endorsing them.[27] Political activist Phyllis Schlafly accused Koop of promoting "safe sodomy and safe fornication," and told him that, rather than inform her own children about condoms, she would rather let "promiscuous young people catch and transmit AIDS."[28] Schlafly's thinking paralleled that of seventeenth-century medical writers who refused to disclose cures for syphilis. The logic was simple: sex outside of marriage, they believed, should never be made safe, even if it could be. Illicit sex carried its own punishment in the form of venereal disease; to make it less dangerous was to subvert the plan of nature—and of nature's God.

Most simply and bluntly, California congressman William Dannemeyer offered his own AIDS prevention strategy to the surgeon general: if it were up to him, Dannemeyer announced, he would simply wipe every HIV-positive individual off the face of the earth.[29]

More pervasive and powerful than these attacks were the indifference and denial that greeted the report in many quarters. The Southern Baptists, for example—the largest Protestant denomination in the United States—decided not to make the report available to their members because it discussed sex outside of marriage.[30] Whether out of moral concern or simply out of disinterest, most Americans went along with the Baptists in this regard. Fifty-one percent of the American public, pollsters determined, did not bother to read the report; among them was President Reagan.[31]

How did Koop react to these responses? In part he was disappointed and puzzled; in part he was angry. As a person of faith, he had tried to find common ground with other believers, and could not understand why he found himself standing on an island rather than an isthmus. "I sometimes feel sorry," he reflected, "for the religious beliefs people have built for themselves that don't have any basis." Particularly incomprehensible to him was the Catholic opposition to condoms: "It stretches the imagination," he admitted.

Koop's skepticism hardened into disdain when he discussed those who had attacked him. Conservatives who had cheered his nomination but turned their backs on him after the AIDS report, he felt, had abandoned "their core beliefs of integrity and compassion." This group included the White House. The president, Koop felt, was competent to understand the ramifications of the epidemic, and could well have handled it more effectively; instead, however, he let his advisers handle *him*. To Koop, such behavior was simply wrong.

Was there a paradox in Koop's role as a conservative Christian who went far out of his way to teach Americans how to have safer sex? The surgeon general believed that it was his duty to protect human lives, whether those of unborn children or those of drug users. Following the centuries-old tradition of Christian healing, Koop saw himself as "the Surgeon General of homosexuals as well as of heterosexuals, and of the promiscuous as well as the moral." Koop's blend of conservative and liberal sentiments recalled that of the seventeenth-century English Dr. L. S., the author of *Prophylaktikon,* who endorsed shipping syphilitic prostitutes off to remote colonial plantations, but who also insisted, with surprising compassion, that "the more loathsome the disease, the more commiseration is required, and the physician is obliged to a more tender care."

Some of Koop's behavior in the AIDS crisis is open to question—in particular, his five years of early silence. Far more than any other member of the Reagan administration, however, he helped to teach America how to overcome its taboos in order to prevent the spread of AIDS. As surgeon general, he helped bring AIDS into the mainstream of public discourse, so that people could see it as something other than a moral scourge wielded by the religious right. As James Curran, for years one of the CDC's leading AIDS researchers and now dean of the School of Public Health at Emory University, put it, reflecting on Koop's role in early years of the epidemic, "He certainly surprised me. He [became] a hero of mine; he was a hero of the times."[32]

STIFLING CANDID MATERIALS

If a single warning about AIDS could have inoculated the country against the new disease, perhaps the surgeon general's report would have sufficed. Like any other public health issue, however—such as stopping smoking, promoting seat-belt use, or encouraging people to eat better and stay fit—effective AIDS prevention required not just a single caution but a continuous campaign, and, unfortunately, each new effort provoked the same old objections. Radicals and moralists were constantly at odds over what was appropriate to say and to show in discussing routes of transmission and acceptable alternatives, and the result was that effective prevention materials often were not produced and distributed—especially when federal funding was involved.

One hugely important battle over prevention materials was started by a single pamphlet published by the Gay Men's Health Crisis of New York. Most GMHC brochures were targeted at adult gay and lesbian readers, and followed the approved public health strategy of portraying safer sex in as positive, upbeat, and erotic a light as possible. GMHC's publications, counseling, and support groups taught gay and bisexual men how to use condoms for anal intercourse, how to kiss, lick, and suck their partners' bodies without exchanging infectious fluids, and how to enjoy activities like voyeurism, masturbation, talking dirty, using sex toys, and watching X-rated videos; intravenous drug users were taught to exchange old needles for new ones and clean their works with bleach if they were shared. Any activity, more or less, was fine, as long as it did not transmit HIV. (Knowing that this approach was controversial, GMHC carefully segregated its funding: public money went to activities acceptable to government agencies, while more controversial projects were paid for by money from private sources.) Within the gay community, GMHC's safer-sex campaigns were generally well regarded. Elsewhere, however, this was not always the case.

One day in October 1987, Senator Jesse Helms marched into the Oval Office with a small brochure in his hand. The pamphlet in question was "After the Gym," part of GMHC's *Safer Sex Comix* series; in it, two muscular male characters named Julio and Ed safely but unabashedly worked off the excitement produced by working out. "Mr. President," declared the senator, "I don't want to ruin your day, but I feel obliged to hand you this and let you look at what is being distributed under the pretense of AIDS education material." Even more shocking than the comic book itself, Helms proclaimed to Reagan, was the fact that GMHC had "received over $600,000 in federal funds from your Administration."[33]

As more than one newspaper would soon report, the president "opened the book, looked at a couple of pages, closed it, shook his head, and hit his desk with his fist," and this thud was soon echoed around the nation. "After the Gym" was just what the nation's conservatives had been looking for: proof that the fight against AIDS was just another way gays and lesbians had found to advance the "homosexual agenda." To Helms and others, "After the Gym" was the worst kind of pornography. Not only did it show people participating in unspeakable acts—it also encouraged its readers to follow the characters' example.[34]

The *Lebanon (Pa.) Daily News* denounced the brochure as "disgusting"; the *Washington Times* found it "more than a bit shocking to ordinary sensibilities." "YUK!" proclaimed the *Minneapolis Daily American*, warning its readers that "gay activists aren't noble crusaders combating a dread disease: they're power-hungry radicals seeking politically-mandated acceptance of their deviant life-style."[35] In an article entitled "Should Our Taxes Promote Safe Sodomy?" syndicated columnist James Kilpatrick revived the notion that those whose diseases resulted from illicit sex were anything but innocent victims. "One can weep for the children," Kilpatrick mused, "but it is hard to work up much sympathy for the sodomists and addicts who have brought the disease upon themselves."[36] Not one to restrict himself to words alone, Helms turned his indignation into action. "Every Christian ethic," he proclaimed on the Senate floor, "cries out for me to do something." An enormous spending bill was lumbering through the chamber at the time—$129 billion worth of funding to support the federal departments of Labor, Health and Human Services, and Education for the entire 1988 fiscal year. To this liberal-proof behemoth, Helms attached a small but highly strategic amendment designed to prevent the federal government from paying for any AIDS education or prevention materials that would "promote or encourage, directly or indirectly, homosexual sexual activities." What American politician could refuse to promote such things? The amendment rolled through the Senate with a 94–2 majority, carried the House 358–47, and became the law of the land.[37]

This small piece of legislative verbiage had an enormous impact on the American AIDS scene. HHS not only published a great deal of AIDS prevention literature itself, but also funded much of what came from state and local health departments. The Helms amendment

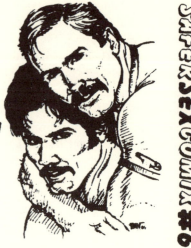

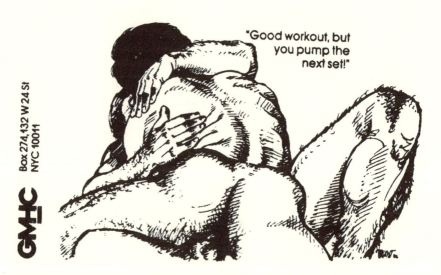

"After the Gym." *Safer Sex Comix* no. 6 (New York: Gay Men's Health Crisis, ca. 1986). © 1986 Gay Men's Health Crisis.

effectively censored the large majority of publicly funded AIDS prevention literature throughout the United States, and its language was so broad that it was not just homoerotic pieces like "After the Gym" that were banned: even a mention of anal intercourse, for example, could be seen as violating the federal mandate.

Fearful of biting the congressional hand that fed it, the CDC immediately adopted strict guidelines that applied to every pamphlet, flier, and poster it printed or paid for. The agency said "no," for example, to any picture of the genital organs, the anus, and either safe *or* unsafe sex.[38] In addition, all prevention materials had to warn about the dangers of promiscuity and IV drug use and propound the benefits of abstinence.[39]

To enforce its rules the CDC set up program review panels—groups of ordinary citizens empowered to ensure that AIDS prevention materials did not violate community norms of decency or taste. The panels followed their mandate scrupulously. In North Carolina, for example, a panel prohibited as "offensive" any reference to sexual orientation; a panel in Los Angeles turned down a poster showing a black man simply *sitting next to* a white man. The words "fun," "exciting," and "sexy" had to be deleted from brochures; so did anything "tacky," "unpatriotic," or "in bad taste." One panel decreed that no information at all on safer sex practices should be included in a general brochure on AIDS. This board of citizens, apparently, felt that it was appropriate to encourage people to avoid a disease, but inappropriate to tell them how.

The Helms amendment flew in the face of AIDS prevention principles endorsed by leading pubic health authorities. The National Academy of Sciences, for example, directed that AIDS prevention materials should contain "explicit, practical, and perhaps graphic advice targeted at specific audiences."[40] The dean of the Harvard School of Public Health, a study by a faculty member at the Mount Sinai School of Medicine, and the *American Journal of Public Health* all strongly endorsed accurate, explicit, and even erotic communication about safer sex, free from moral censure.[41] Failure to follow these principles carried grave risks, authorities warned: the highly prestigious Institute of Medicine cautioned that "efforts to stifle candid materials may take a toll in human lives."

The conflict between CDC guidelines and public health principles posed substantial practical problems for public health agencies. Designing an AIDS prevention brochure for readers with little education, for example, the Red Cross confronted a dilemma: whether to use the colloquial term "cum," which the CDC rules prohibited, or the acceptable but (to some) meaninglessly clinical "semen." "We were thus faced with two bad choices," worried the agency: "to leave the [slang] term in and not have the brochure approved for distribution by some states' program review panels, including California, or to replace it with a word the audience did not understand."[42]

In an effort to change the national rules, GMHC took the Department of Health and Human Services to court. Limiting public funds for AIDS prevention, GMHC argued, guaranteed that the underprivileged would fail to get the information they needed to protect themselves. People who could pay private doctors, or who had special-interest groups dedicated to their welfare, could learn how to prevent AIDS from these sources. Those without these advantages, however, had to depend on whatever vague and incomplete information the government saw fit to provide. Like medieval lepers whose families could not care for them at home or place them in hospices, like indigent syphilitics cast out from public hospitals, and like the working-class Londoners who did not have the means to leave the city for their country houses when plague loomed in 1665, the American poor were badly informed about and underprotected against AIDS, and their rates of infection were correspondingly high.

Ostensibly, sex was at issue. In court, however, GMHC argued that its case was really about the morality of life and death. Citing the Reverend Scott Allen of the Texas Baptist General Convention, the agency argued that it was better to produce a brochure someone might find offensive than it was to see a person die from AIDS who might have been spared.[43] Part of the reason that the arguing was so bitter was that each side was convinced it had the truly moral position: one side saw safer sex as the route to health; the other, as the road to hell.

On 11 May 1992, the U.S. District Court in Manhattan found in favor of GMHC: the CDC, the court decided, had exceeded its legal authority, and its content restrictions were unconstitutionally vague. As another court, earlier in the trial, had held, the offensiveness standard was "one of the greatest single handicaps imposed on professional educators who must depend on government funding for their AIDS-related educational efforts."[44] GMHC had won the right for AIDS prevention to take priority over parochial views—but only after years of effort. There is no way to know precisely how many Americans died as a result of the Helms amendment and the CDC's content restrictions, but the numbers are likely to have been substantial. Hundreds of thousands of Americans were probably infected with HIV between 1988 and 1992. Could effective education have prevented 10 percent of these infections? 5 percent? Even if only one infection in a hundred could have been averted, the cost of sparing the country's moral sensibilities ranked in the thousands of lives.

A CARDINAL SIN

Much of the furor over the surgeon general's report and the Helms amendment was linked with America's Protestant heritage, but the Catholic Church played a substantial role in the American AIDS crisis as well. Many Catholic responses to AIDS were strongly positive, particularly in the area of medical care: St. Vincent's and St. Clare's Hospitals in New York, for example, provided entire wards dedicated to those with the disease, and Mother Teresa set a model for Catholic compassion toward the sick, both in India and in her visits to the United States. The fact that AIDS was sexually transmitted and that many of the principles of safer sex conflicted absolutely with Church teachings, however, made it extremely difficult for Catholic institutions and theologians to get on board the prevention train. These conflicts showed up in a history of jagged inconsistencies and, sometimes, very public fights.

Between the Middle Ages and the twentieth century, Catholic theology evolved in many ways, but it remained remarkably conservative in regard to sex. Medieval penitential manuals had been particularly stringent about such sexual misdeeds as fornication, homosexuality, adultery, and masturbation, and these prohibitions remained in force in modern times. Even as the third millennium approached, celibacy continued to be the only acceptable pattern of life for members of the Catholic clergy. Only in regard to sex within marriage did changes come, and these were slow and limited: until the twentieth century, the Church still held that sex between husband and wife was sinful unless it was redeemed by procreation. After World War I, however, in an encyclical entitled *Chaste Spouses* (*Casti connubii*), Pope Pius XI finally declared that marriage existed not only to produce Christian offspring, but also to bind married couples to God "through Christian love and mutual support." Hidden in the foliage of this inconspicuous phrase was the novel idea that sex and love in and of themselves had value within Christian marriage.[45]

This liberalization, however, did not extend very far. Abortion and any kind of contraception, for example, remained strictly forbidden.[46] With birth control, declared Pope John Paul II, even marital sex was sex for pleasure only, and thus a sin: following a tradition more than a thousand years old, he declared it "adultery in the heart." For John Paul, the body was something that good Catholics should govern "like a compliant tool."[47]

The Church was no more tolerant toward homosexuality than it was toward abortion. Vatican II, the Second Vatican Council of 1962–1965, had provided a few liberal glimmerings in this area, but these did not have a widespread effect: much more typical was the view propounded in a 1960s Catholic treatise on natural law that explained that "it is clear from sex duality what forms of sexual behavior are in conformity with nature, and what forms are not."[48] Penises belonged in vaginas and in wedlock, and nowhere else. In a 1986 letter, Cardinal Joseph Ratzinger, John Paul's theological watchdog, reluctantly acknowledged that homosexual orientation was not a sin per se, but he warned all concerned that it was "a more or less strong tendency ordered toward an intrinsic moral evil," and that the gay rights movement was nothing but "deceitful propaganda."[49] If secular governments decided to pass laws supporting homosexuality, the cardinal warned, they were violating the very order of nature, and "neither the Church nor society at large should be surprised when . . . irrational and violent reactions increase."[50] Nature violated, in other words, would return the injury that had been done to her.

In light of these views, it was a major surprise when, in December 1987, the Catholic bishops of the United States gave qualified support to the idea of teaching that condoms could prevent the spread of AIDS. In fact, most of what the bishops had to say in this declaration was hardly radical, or even particularly tolerant. They maintained that Christ's teachings about sexuality were absolute truths; they insisted that all people should live chaste lives; and they claimed that AIDS was spreading through the world because "some people will not act as they can and should." They also squarely stated that no sex outside of marriage could possibly be "safe." Nevertheless, like Surgeon General Koop, they acknowledged that they lived in a pluralistic society, and in a world in which both HIV and prophylactics played a role. Under these circumstances, the bishops cautiously proposed, it might be acceptable for public health authorities to teach about condoms and safer sex in their efforts to prevent AIDS.[51] "This reflects a pastoral acknowledgment of the real world," marveled a Loyola University theologian to a reporter. "You don't often find that in [Church] statements connected with human sexuality."[52]

Episcopal traditionalists were equally surprised by the letter, but far less pleased. "There's no such thing as safe, or safer sex," declared Archbishop John Mahony of Los Angeles: "that's an illusion." Archbishop Anthony Bevilacqua of Pittsburgh announced that he was "strongly opposed to passing out condoms under any circumstances." And New York's Cardinal John J. O'Connor capped the discussion with a typically pointed remark: "The use of condoms is immoral in a pluralistic society or any other society," he declared.[53] As far as these prelates were concerned, the Church had the right to impose its views on sexual morality not just on Catholics, but on all.

Faced with such strident rebukes, the bishops issued a hasty retraction. The revised statement—ratified by a vote of 219 to 4—declared contritely that safer sex was *not* the moral equivalent of abstinence, expressed concern that the safer-sex approach to prevention might lure many into promiscuity, and warned that AIDS would not stop spreading until people lived their sexual lives in accordance with what the Church saw as "authentic, human values"—namely, abstinence and monogamous, heterosexual marriage. "Casual sex is a threat to health," the bishops declared, implying that AIDS was a likely, even inevitable, consequence of straying from the straight and narrow path, and stating with finality that "it is not condom use that is the solution to this health problem."[54] In the official Catholic view, as in the view of other groups like the Texas-based Medical Institute for Sexual Health, AIDS was fundamentally a moral, not a medical problem, and so could not be resolved by medical means.[55] As the Catholic journal *Human Life International Reports* bluntly put it a few months later, "The use of condoms protects the users neither from Hell nor from AIDS."[56]

With this declaration, the bishops brought one of the most fundamental AIDS issues to the surface: was it a sickness, or was it God's or nature's punishment for sexual sins? Approaches to AIDS prevention rode largely on this question. Those who believed that AIDS was primarily or exclusively a medical issue focused their efforts on keeping the virus from spreading. For them, it scarcely mattered whether sex was hetero- or homosexual, whether it occurred inside or outside of marriage, whether intercourse was vaginal or anal—as long as it was protected. For religious traditionalists, on the other hand, AIDS was the inevitable and perhaps even proper result of sexual sin. God had decreed, nature had revealed, and religion had propounded the proper uses of sexuality; anything else was wrong and therefore dangerous. The idea that a rubber prophylactic could render anal intercourse between two men safe, for example, would be laughable were the consequences not so deadly. The terms of the debate, mutatis mutandis, were not all that different from the thirteenth-century controversy over lovesickness and the coital cure. Was it acceptable to prevent a fatal illness by committing a mortal sin? The medieval Church and its most conservative American successors answered unanimously: no. Humanity's duty to God was to behave according to the dictates of Catholic virtue. If people died in the process, the loss of life was regrettable, but ultimately less catastrophic than the loss of souls.

MURDER IN THE CATHEDRAL

Not everyone, of course, agreed with this position, particularly in what the bishops had briefly recognized as a pluralistic society—a society of which New York City was a prime example. There were many reasons why this city was the center of many of the cultural battles in the AIDS wars. One was that New York City and New York State had the largest AIDS caseload in the nation, especially early on. By the end of December 1987, for example, over 120,000 cases had been reported in adults and children in New York State—five-sixths of these in the city.[57] An additional factor was that many of the major figures in the national debate about AIDS were based there, including GMHC, ACT-UP, and Cardinal O'Connor, just to name a few. And another was New York City itself. Bound together by a huge, dense population, the biggest mass transit system in the country, and an intense concentration of media, New York was a community in which few local events were denied their full share of attention. In the nuclear holocaust of the American AIDS crisis, New York was, as gay writer Andrew Holleran put it, ground zero.

It was not altogether surprising, therefore, that New York's Cardinal John J. O'Connor should have been the nation's loudest Catholic voice on AIDS. A former navy chaplain and a Georgetown Ph.D., O'Connor (born in Philadelphia in 1920) was named Archbishop of New York in 1983 and became cardinal the following year. Vocal on many issues and fond of amplifying his sentiments through skilful use of the tabloid press, O'Connor attained national prominence with his stands on abortion, homosexuality, and AIDS,[58] and as a result was named to the Reagan Commission on AIDS in 1987 and gave the opening address at the Vatican conference on AIDS in 1989. Loudly and consistently, the cardinal articulated a strong and simple message about the epidemic: that no matter what anyone else might say, traditional sexual morality was the only solution to the crisis. Sometimes he delivered this message in a positive tone: "Good morality is good medicine," he would announce, urging single Americans to remain celibate and married ones to remain chaste.[59] Sometimes he sounded like a knowing and perceptive coach, reminding his team that prophylactics were out of bounds. By distributing condoms, he explained, "you bring all of society down. You're saying that we lost the ball game. You're saying that people can't be educated, you can't appeal to their better natures."[60] And sometimes he recalled the centuries-old voice of the Franciscan monk Michel Menot, who had warned his congregants in his Lenten sermons in 1508 that syphilis—as new then as AIDS was in the 1980s—simply worked the will of God: "Lust shortens the days of mankind," Menot had preached. Centuries later, a similar warning came from Cardinal O'Connor: "Don't blame the Church," he warned, "if people get a disease because they violate Church teaching."[61] Christ and his church had offered humankind a straight path to safety and salvation, the cardinal believed; woe would befall those who turned aside.

Pronouncements like this made O'Connor a natural lightning rod for the ire of AIDS radicals, and so it was no surprise that St. Patrick's Cathedral—O'Connor's seat—was the venue for a protest that occurred just two weeks after the bishops' revised letter was made public. On Sunday, 10 December 1989, hundreds of ACT-UP protesters mingled with the crowds of worshipers and inconspicuously filtered into the cathedral; meanwhile, other demonstrators surrounded the building with protest signs. Inside, as the cardinal was saying mass, some ACT-UP members dropped silently to the ground in an AIDS "die-in"; one protestor symbolically broke a communion wafer and hurled it to the flagstone floor. Others disrupted the service by standing and shouting "You bigot, O'Connor, you're killing us!" Overwhelmed by the chaos, the cardinal slumped in his seat and covered his face with his hands.[62]

One hundred eleven protestors were arrested that Sunday, and in the following week a national uproar took place as politicians and the media proclaimed their fierce disapproval of the action. A coalition of moderate gay and lesbian groups condemned ACT-UP for violating the Bill of Rights; the right-wing New York Post declared that a sacrilege had occurred, and took advantage of the opportunity to endorse the cardinal's "good morality is good medicine" policy. New York's liberal Democratic mayor, David Dinkins, deplored the episode; vice president Dan Quayle called it "outrageous."[63] Taking heart, the cardinal reconsecrated the cathedral and, in passing, reiterated the Church's view that "homosexuality is sinful, until the end of time."[64]

In terms of public relations, the cardinal emerged from the battle ahead of ACT-UP. In terms of AIDS prevention, however, this incident did nothing so much as to reveal the breadth of the gap between the two opposing sides of the issue. As National Institutes of Health historian Victoria Harden recalls, both camps "viewed each other as political enemies and attempted to manipulate the political system to support their positions. Each also tried (but not very hard, I think) to win the hearts and votes of the great middle group that didn't feel so strongly about the issues."[65] Among the major players, the stakes had risen too high for compromise; the theatrics of the confrontations left little common ground, and did little to promote policies that would benefit the public health.

The incident at St. Patrick's was largely symbolic, but the issues it represented were often intensely pragmatic ones. Governments, hospitals, and agencies had to decide what they were going to do to educate the public about HIV, which prevention strategies to employ, and how they would deal with the needs of the sick and those at risk for infection. The same principles and characters that had collided at the cathedral ran into one another wherever AIDS policy was formed and AIDS prevention programs enacted. Here again, the same questions arose that had haunted the response to lovesickness, leprosy, syphilis, plague, and masturbation: was it a sickness, or was it the result of sin? As in the past, these conflicts were played out on the bodies of the vulnerable and the ill.

One place in which these bodies turned up was the wards of the city's Catholic hospitals. In New York, as around the country, the medieval Catholic tradition of providing medical care in hospitals remained strong in the late twentieth century, and Catholic hospitals provided some of the best and most compassionate care available to patients, including patients with AIDS. In the area of sexual health, however, Catholic institutions parted company from their secular counterparts: they were forbidden to perform abortions, provide counseling on contraception—or teach AIDS patients about safer sex.[66]

By the late 1980s, New York's AIDS caseload was growing so rapidly that the city was running short of hospital beds for the sick. Motivated partly by the desire to provide care, and partly (argued GMHC's former associate executive director Michael Isbell) by the state's exceptionally high reimbursements for AIDS care, the Catholic hospitals offered to build wards to accommodate the overload.[67] The sticking point, however, was that, to prevent the continuing spread of infection, the state required its health care providers to counsel their patients on safer sex. This Cardinal O'Connor flatly refused to let his hospitals do.

Here the twin doctrinal imperatives of offering care and maintaining sexual orthodoxy came into combat, and the cardinal—perhaps unwittingly—revealed this conflict. On the one hand, O'Connor portrayed himself as a compassionate caregiver. "I have sat with, listened to, wiped the lesions of, prayed with, or emptied the bedpans of more than one thousand persons with AIDS," he declared—a claim that may have been less than literally true.[68] At the same time, he ridiculed the techniques that public health authorities endorsed for stopping the spread of HIV. "In order to get AIDS money to facilities run by nuns," he announced, "they will have to teach the residents there to masturbate and also show them obscene films."[69] The fact of the matter, however, was that safer-sex instruction had been endorsed by many major public health authorities, and these requirements came from the same source as the money with which the cardinal wanted to expand his hospitals.

Some public figures, such as New York's governor Mario Cuomo, ignored the problem; others, such as city council member Thomas Duane, decried it. Gay legal authority Thomas B. Stoddard, head of the Lambda Legal Defense Fund and a professor at NYU Law School, denounced the state's willingness to cooperate with the archdiocese on this issue as "unhealthy if not unconstitutional."[70] Officially, the decision went in the cardinal's favor: the state provided its funds and looked discreetly away from the prevention problems. Unofficially, however, the Catholic hospitals made some tacit compromises of their own. At times, the cardinal would be holding forth in one room at St. Vincent's while the hospital's medical staff surreptitiously handed out condoms in the next.[71] Such behavior may have saved face, but it did nothing to address, and little to resolve, the philosophical differences that pervaded AIDS policy in the city, the state, and the nation.

Schoolhouse Blues

The most critical prevention battles were fought not in hospitals but in high schools and elementary schools, where the future of the epidemic would be determined: even nine-year-olds, after all, were only a few years away from puberty, and with it the risk of infection. American teenagers were not more sexually active than their European counterparts, but in part because the country was so reluctant to educate its young people about sex, the United States had more cases of sexually transmitted disease than any other nation in the developed world. Through the late 1990s, more than twelve million Americans a year developed STDs—the most common infections in America—and three million of these were teenagers, who far surpassed adults in the numbers subject to chlamydia, pelvic inflammatory disease, and human papilloma virus.[72] Religious teens were not exempt from sexual activity and its risks: a 1984 study of 10,000 "churched adolescents" showed that 9 percent of seventh-grade girls and 22 percent of seventh-grade boys stated that they had already had sexual intercourse.[73] Even more disturbing, some sources estimated that one girl in four was sexually abused before she turned eighteen.[74] The need for AIDS prevention among young Americans was overwhelming.

Public health authorities from Surgeon General Koop to the World Health Organization urged that children be taught HIV basics from the elementary years, adjusting the curriculum to the students' level of understanding. Most of the nation supported this position. In a 1990 study, Harvard School of Public Health professor Robert Blendon found that 94 percent of Americans supported AIDS education in public schools. Eight out of ten believed this instruction should begin in grade school; just as many wanted it to include talk of prophylactics. Almost all thought that children should have been taught about condoms by the end of middle school.[75]

This apparent consensus, however, did not guarantee smooth sailing for an AIDS curriculum. Any issue that linked sex and disease with children—as the old masturbation scares had shown—created panic. The issues about AIDS education that had caused trouble in Congress and in New York's Catholic hospitals created huge obstacles to effective AIDS prevention in classrooms and school board meetings all across the country. Thus, in 1990, the State of Connecticut appropriated $7 million to its Drug Free Schools program, but only $297,000—less than one-twentieth as much money—to prevent the transmission of HIV.[76]

The thought of AIDS instruction terrorized parents. "YOU CAN'T TAKE OUR KIDS!" screamed a 1993 New York Post ad placed by the Guardian Family Association. "We are fearful," the fine print confessed, "of new AIDS curriculums that teach children as young as the fourth grade graphic details of anal, oral, and vaginal sex."[77] Similarly, in 1996, parents in Chappaqua, New York, barred Magic Johnson's AMA-approved book about AIDS from their schools: the lessons it taught, the parents felt, were too explicit for their children to learn. (Spreading their sexual concerns to other diseases as well, the same parents also found it indecent to teach young people how to examine themselves for breast and testicular cancer.[78]) The specter of childhood sexuality dictated school-based AIDS education policy in the 1990s, regardless of the dangers that ignorance held. These fears led twenty-six states to mandate abstinence programs for their schools—even though these programs had never been proven to reduce teen sex.[79] Beliefs about innocence and guilt, sex and sin, that affected the history of sexually transmitted diseases for centuries proved still to be powerful persuaders when American parents decided what their children should and should not learn.

Some of the loudest protests on this subject came from the Catholic hierarchy, and these did not always remain focused on the religious side of the church-state divide. In 1989, for example, Cardinal Bernard Law of Boston told Catholic parents to keep their children out of AIDS classes in public schools, citing the lessons' "moral and physical danger."[80] In 1992, the Bishop of Brooklyn managed to pressure New York State officials to withdraw from circulation among *public school* teachers 14,000 copies of a guide to AIDS education the bishop considered inappropriate.[81] The following year, the superintendent of New York's Catholic school system urged that the city's public schools be purged of "secularism and hedonism." "Purge the system of secularism?" exclaimed an astonished *New York Newsday* columnist. "It's a secular school system!"[82] As with the debate over the bishops' letter and the pluralism of American society, the Church hierarchy often saw itself as a moral arbiter for Catholics and non-Catholics alike.

One of the more explosive fights occurred in New York, where the quest for an AIDS curriculum led to the ouster of a chancellor of the schools. In 1990, the city hired Miami schools superintendent Joseph Fernandez to run the public school system, whose problems included a high dropout rate, a decaying infrastructure, and an oversized central bureaucracy.[83] What ultimately brought Fernandez down, however, was not these issues but the debate over condoms and sex education.

Fernandez had good reason to be concerned. Four out of five New York City students, a 1990 study by the Alan Guttmacher Institute found, had had sexual intercourse by the age of nineteen. Pregnancy and STD rates were correspondingly high: 128 per thousand fourteen- to nineteen-year-olds were pregnant in 1989, and New York had more cases of adolescent AIDS than any other city in the country. Fernandez wrote in his memoir that "the school system has a moral responsibility to its children. Its children were dying, and although many would die no matter what we did, if we did nothing the numbers would be apocalyptic. Somebody had to take a position of leadership, so why not the schools?"[84] The Board of Education, however, did not share the chancellor's concern. The board did narrowly pass a condom availability plan in 1991, but the opposition was implacable: two members, in fact, threatened to take the matter to court. Meanwhile, the chancellor created an additional brouhaha when he suspended a school board in Queens that had declared his new Rainbow Curriculum to be "aimed at promoting acceptance of sodomy" and "shot through with dangerously misleading homosexual propaganda."[85]

The long battle ended with a contentious Board of Education meeting on 10 February 1993, at which one protestor, carried away by religious vehemence, shouted, "Mr. Fernandez is a devil!"[86] In the end, the board decided to let the chancellor go. The following Sunday morning, Cardinal O'Connor used his sermon at St. Patrick's to congratulate the Board of Education members who had voted Fernandez out.[87] Once again, religious and moral conservatives felt that it was their right—if not their obligation—to influence health policy for all the children and parents of the city of New York. As on the national front, sectarian views of morality outweighed the protection of public health.

Sodom on the Subway

The fighting over safer-sex prevention programs continued on many fronts across the country, but this chapter will examine only one more—another episode in New York City history in which the religious right and the gay left carried out an ultrapublic argument over the morality and the science of safer sex. In this case, both sides attempted to convert the public to their views, and here both sides lost—the AIDS activists because they forgot a crucial element of their strategy, the conservatives because they abandoned the truth.

On 14 January 1994, GMHC began a new prevention campaign called "Young, Hot, and Safe." Following its success in eroticizing safer sex for adults, the agency decided to use the same approach with teenagers, placing provocative ads in the city's subway cars. The rationale behind this move was that the public venue would attract attention to the campaign, but this was also the plan's greatest flaw. In using such a broad-spectrum approach, GMHC neglected a critical point it had made again and again in its case against the CDC: that although offensiveness was not necessarily a first consideration, AIDS prevention messages had to be specifically focused on their target audiences. The target of "Young, Hot, and Safe"—sexually active teenagers—was certainly a part of the public that saw the ads, but so were all kinds of other people, many of whom were less than happy to have these reminders confront them on their daily ride to work.

Less than a week after the billboards appeared, a public outcry arose. The *New York Post* decried the ads as "sleazy and outrageous," "recruiting posters for teenage promiscuity" that ignored the only effective strategy for preventing AIDS—that of just saying no.[88] The *Daily News* agreed: for the young and unmarried, it argued, sex was always a risk: "Why not just change the words 'young, hot, and safe' to 'young, foolish, and dead'?" The Diocese of Brooklyn seconded this opinion. These ads, the diocese declared, were part of GMHC's "calculated campaign to have the homosexual lifestyle put on a par with normal family living." GMHC, pointing out that New York State adolescent AIDS cases had increased by 222 percent over the previous five years, responded that "life in an epidemic changes the rules." At least one neighborhood paper, *Our Town*, supported this position, deriding the conservatives as ostriches and proclaiming "'Family Values' Won't Save Our Youth."[89]

The next turn of events showed how deeply the conservatives had been offended and the lengths to which they were prepared to go to get their views to the public. On 26 April, the Catholic League announced that it would post 2,500 proabstinence ads in the trains to "retaliate" for GMHC's winter campaign, which, the league claimed, was "not warranted medically or morally." The ads read,

> Want to know a dirty little secret?
> CONDOMS DON'T SAVE LIVES.
> But restraint does.
>> Only fools think condoms are foolproof.
>> Remember, better safe than sorry.
>>> —*Some common sense and a public service message*
>>> *from the Catholic League for Religious and Civil Rights*

Here, the league was taking liberties with the truth. Condoms were not foolproof, but they did save lives; the problem with condoms, for the most part, was not that the devices were faulty but that people used them inconsistently or incorrectly.[90] People made these mistakes for a variety of reasons. Some people didn't like the feel of sex with a prophylactic; others were overconfident that they or their partners were disease-free. Some felt guilty or embarrassed about using condoms, or about having sex at all. And others trusted misleading information spread around by those who believed that using a condom was a sin. As recently as 1991, for example, only 26 percent of Americans believed that condoms were "very effective" in preventing the spread of AIDS.[91] By saying over and over again that condoms did not work, the antiprophylactic forces contributed to an environment in which, in fact, they did not.

Public health authorities were quick to attack the "Dirty Little Secret" campaign, which city health commissioner Margaret Hamburg condemned as "scientifically untrue." The dean of the Columbia School of Public Health denounced the league's blitz as "a major public health disaster"; the education director of the American Foundation for AIDS Research, herself an ordained minister, condemned it as "absolutely, unequivocally misleading."[92] In its zeal to contradict GMHC, the Catholic League had abandoned its claims to public trust, and its ads were eventually pulled. Once again, a battle over AIDS prevention had left the public confused and at risk.

MISTAKES WERE MADE

America was hardly the only country in the world in which prejudice, parochialism, and fear created public policy disasters in the face of AIDS. No country on the planet is now free from HIV, and each nation's experiences with the disease reflect the weak points in its thinking, planning, and compassion. In most nations, the poor are, as always, disproportionately affected. Often women—whether wives, girlfriends, or prostitutes—are exposed without the ability to protect themselves. In the United States in the 1990s, a new face of AIDS had emerged. Many American gay men who had survived the first wave paid more attention to the lessons of prevention, but other disenfranchised classes—younger gay men, drug addicts, African and Latino Americans, and women—donned the burning mantle of the disease. In centralized, highly bureaucratic France and Japan, hundreds of people were needlessly infected when their governments refused to incur the costs of withdrawing infected blood from the national supply. The list goes on and on. But it is fair to say that, for a country of its economic and medical resources, America was substantially less effective at confronting this threat to national health and security than it should have been.

There have been some AIDS success stories. Australia and the sexually pragmatic Scandinavian countries, for example, have had relatively effective prevention efforts; one Dutch researcher estimated, in 1995, that the rate of HIV infection in the Netherlands was about one-third that of the United States. Even countries with huge obstacles confronting them, such as war-torn Uganda, and Thailand with its pervasive sex industry, have made significant national steps in preventing AIDS.[93] Ideally, the United States might have been a member of this group.

There are innumerable reasons why America did not do better at preventing the spread of this epidemic. One was that the virus came early to American shores, and spread quickly and silently for years before anyone was really aware of it. "By the time there were ten thousand cases of AIDS in the United States," Emory public health school dean

James Curran pointed out, "there were four hundred thousand people infected. . . . In San Francisco, by the time the first cases of AIDS were reported, thirty percent of the gay men in the city were infected." Another was that, for years, many homosexual men viewed gay rights as inseparable from the freedom to have sex as often as possible, and with few, if any, constraints. Many of us were appallingly slow to recognize that this freedom could in fact be dangerous—that there were risks, as well as benefits, to liberalizing sexual *mores.* This liberty-at-all-costs philosophy gained ground in the mid-1990s with the public emergence of "barebacking"—practicing anal sex without condoms, as author Gabriel Rotello pointed out in his 1997 book *Sexual Ecology.* Openly gay men, according to studies Rotello cited, participated in riskier sexual activity than closeted or bisexual men—at least in part because they often had sex while high on drugs or alcohol, factors present in 60 percent of unsafe encounters—and in part because their subcultures promoted unsafe sex.[94] (Rotello was also correct in noting, however, that the nation's elevated abortion rates showed America's heterosexuals to be scarcely more careful about unprotected sex than gay men.) Other reasons for the continued spread of the epidemic included the enormous and unconscionable gaps in the American health care system, and the fact that—as Curran observed—American physicians were not oriented toward disease prevention. The myriad vagaries of human nature, and the physical, emotional, and spiritual fatigue among affected communities after nearly twenty years of pervasive sickness and death also played their part. Prevention is a lifetime issue, as Curran and Dr. Helene Gayle, director of the National Center for HIV, STD, and TB Prevention at the CDC, have stated, but this was not something that most people truly understood, accepted, and put into practice.

Another major cause for America's failure to prevent the spread of HIV, of course, was the great national anxiety about sex and the widespread prevalence of the age-old attitudes this book has traced. Public figures like Jerry Falwell, Jesse Helms, and John O'Connor did not create these fears and prejudices: they merely reawakened beliefs that had held power for thousands of years. Growing from religious roots, these ideas spread luxuriantly over the fertile soil of the American popular mind. Throughout the first half-dozen years of the epidemic they gained in popularity and strength, shaping policies in Washington and attitudes at the mall. Those who saw AIDS as God's punishment for homosexuality were the heirs to centuries of preachers, physicians, and ordinary people who believed that disease was God's way of responding to human sin, and, in particular, to sins involving sex. The Fourth

Lateran Council, decreeing in 1215 that doctors were not to reveal the coital cure to their lovesick patients; the religious and secular authorities who stood medieval lepers in open graves, annulled their marriages, and expelled them from hospices for any hint of sexual activity; the hospitals and towns that barred their gates to syphilitics, and the physicians who shut them up in mercury-vapor steam baths till their teeth fell out and their systems were poisoned; the preachers who saw plague as a broom with which God swept the most nasty and uncomely corners of the universe and the officials who decreed that the bodies of the plague dead could not be buried among the uninfected in ordinary churchyards; and physicians who cauterized, circumcised, and clitoridectomized the unanesthetized bodies of their masturbating patients—all these found new life in the epidemic that blossomed darkly in American cities in the 1980s. Despite the innumerable changes that had taken place across the centuries, a fear of disease, a need to explain the natural world in human terms, and a lingering uneasiness about sex and sin made it possible for old ideas to take on form, strength, and power. The disease was new, the response was old, and the consequences were disastrous. Not only did the infected and the sick suffer discrimination and shame, but prevention was drastically hindered as well.

Bit by bit, compassion overcame prejudice and fear. Numerous Protestant denominations tried to change public attitudes. In 1986, for example, the Presbyterian Church in the United States was moved to announce that AIDS was not punishment for immoral behavior. Two years later, the Methodist bishops joined the chorus, noting that HIV was not a curse from God; the conservative Moody Bible Institute published a similar view in its newsletter. A gay Protestant movement, the Metropolitan Community Church, reminded the faithful of the example of Jesus, who had explained that a child blind from birth was so afflicted not because of any sin he or his parents had committed, but as an example of God's work. The executive director of a group called Evangelicals for Social Action took specific issue with the Moral Majority on AIDS, arguing that even if homosexuality was a sin, it was no greater a sin than adultery, greed, gossip, racism, or materialism—all common human coin.[95] Clerics who denounced people with AIDS as sinners were harshly taken to task. John Shelby Spong, the Episcopal bishop of Newark, said that the Catholic Church's policies on homosexuals put it "in danger of losing its soul." Rabbi Joseph Edelheit of Chicago, a member of President Clinton's Advisory Council on AIDS, argued that it was not a wrathful god but "clergy who choose doctrine over lives" who would be responsible for AIDS deaths that effective education could have prevented.[96] These rebuttals and denunciations were powerful, but the simple fact that so many of them were deemed necessary revealed the depth and strength of people's religious prejudices about AIDS.

Public figures levied similar criticisms of the American government's response to the epidemic. As early as 1985, Dr. Edward Brandt announced that American public responses to the disease were inadequate. In 1988, the journal *Critical Social Policy* suggested that the American government treated AIDS less as an illness than as a crime, while the National Academy of Sciences blamed the federal government for a lack of guidance. In 1992, June Osborn, M.D., completing her four years as chair of President Bush's National Commission on AIDS, announced that "there really is nothing too hard that can be said about the lack of leadership of the Administration to this epidemic." Retiring after twenty years with the CDC, Don Francis, M.D., declared that he had "never witnessed science abandoned for political principles quite so thoroughly" as it had been in the case of AIDS, and he warned, "A society that allows narrow political vision to guide public health policy is doomed to succumb to disease."[97]

The Clinton administration made good on many of the shortcomings of its predecessors, both in funding and in rhetoric, but some of the same problems remained. Clinton fired surgeon general Joycelyn Elders over AIDS prevention policy differences; he appointed a series of weak and ineffectual "AIDS czars." His first national AIDS strategy—not unveiled until 1996—was characterized by journalists as lacking in any major new initiatives.[98] He was no more effective in preventing the spread of HIV among intravenous drug users, one of the populations that continued to be ravaged by AIDS. Columbia School of Public Health professor Ron Bayer warned that infection through dirty needles would come to be the "dominant wave" of the AIDS epidemic, and Emory's Dean Curran lamented in 1997 that in this area America had made "no progress" since 1981. Needle exchange programs were proven to reduce HIV transmission without increasing drug use, but in 1998 Clinton nonetheless refused to fund them. In a disturbing and hypocritical footnote, a bill passed the House of Representatives in May 1998 to provide "compassionate payments" of $100,000 each to hemophiliacs, their spouses, and their children infected with HIV between 1982 and 1987.[99] The notion of "innocent victims" of AIDS was alive and well funded. No one, however, was passing bills to compensate those infected because the federal government did not provide adequate information on safer sex and intravenous drug use.

Had America done better at preventing the spread of AIDS, it could have saved huge amounts of public and private money;[100] more important, it might have saved countless lives. AIDS has been not only a massive killer, but also a "Rorschach test for Western civilization," and "the biggest and best teacher of the essentials of human life," according to ethicists Richard Smith and Elizabeth Kübler-Ross.[101] The country has learned these lessons only in a spotty and incomplete manner.

Some things America did well. With surprising speed, much of the nation overcame its fear and loathing and developed a persistent and generous compassion. Discrimination against and maltreatment of people with AIDS, though not infrequent, were typically the result of individual prejudice rather than of concerted policies. Despite the urgings of some prominent public figures, notes medical ethicist and MacArthur Fellow Carol Levine, the sick and infected were not tattooed, quarantined, or rounded up into camps.[102] After a shamefully slow start, government-funded research increased, and scientific progress was made. Treatments have improved substantially, and though a vaccine and a cure are not yet within sight, it is not unreasonable to think that they are on the horizon. In every area *except* prevention, Jim Curran argues—protection of the blood supply, surveillance, research—the United States did better than any other country. There is hope.

Even with all these accomplishments and the recent advances in medical treatment, however, CDC epidemiologist Harold Jaffe points out that the real progress against AIDS will be made with condoms that cost a few cents each, not with thousands and thousands of dollars' worth of antiretroviral drugs. Yet the U.S. government's 1992 multibillion dollar, multimedia AIDS prevention campaign could not use the word "condom" or even the word "sex," and three of the four major television networks still refuse to carry condom advertising. Telling teenagers to be abstinent, warning drug users to "just say no," and ignoring homosexuals altogether (the federal government still produces no prevention materials directly aimed at gay men, notes activist Douglas Crimp) virtually guaranteed that more citizens in these groups would die. As the CDC's Gayle observed, the responsibility of the government's public health agencies is to save the lives of *all* citizens, not just of some, yet in this area these agencies have not lived up to their task.

The costs of this epidemic have been enormous. AIDS has killed more than 400,000 Americans—more than died in Korea and Vietnam. A small proportion of these have been people I knew. My loss is minor in comparison to the national tolls, but its effects on my life have been great. Some of the dearest were Michael Botkin (1957–1996), a psychologist, writer, and activist of uncommon learning and sparkling wit; Nick Vance (1958–1994), whose beauty, warmth, and artistic talents helped him to overcome numerous handicaps and brighten many lives; Tom Cunningham (1960–1992), a funny, sweet man who gave a voice to those who had none and came to glory as coordinator of ACT-UP New York; and Tom Stoddard (1949–1997), a humanitarian and teacher who taught me not only about the law, but also about how to find happiness even in a life whose end was nearer than I ever imagined. Another was Stewart Telfer (1955–1990), who was twenty-one when I met him and thirty-four when he died in my arms. Stewart never reconciled his religious beliefs with his sexuality. Perhaps he did not have the strength for this reconciliation; perhaps, as the end came, he cared less about such things than about making his peace with himself and with the people he loved. Perhaps the task of building the bridge was left to me, even though his religion was not mine.

The gap between conservative and activist views of sex and disease has swallowed up too many lives; it is a rift in the bedrock of this nation. Too many of my friends and heroes are dead; too many people are still being infected. I call upon this country to rise up, to remember that we *are* our brothers' and sisters' keepers, and to draw from our faith and experience the strength and compassion we will need to bring an end to this suffering and bring about a future in which there can be love and health enough for all.

CONCLUSION

The Week Nobody Died

What comes after AIDS? It is hard even to ask, let alone to try to answer, that question, when the death tolls and rates of new infection are still rising around the world. And yet, on the day when I began to write this conclusion, I learned that the *Bay Area Reporter*, a gay newspaper in San Francisco, had at last published an issue without an obituary. In that particular community, in that particular corner of the world, there finally came a week in which nobody died. Despite the enormous levels of sickness in Africa and Asia, despite the fact that the latest round of drugs will lose their effectiveness, despite the persistence of new infections in intravenous drug users, their sexual partners, African American and Latina women, and young gay men, the AIDS crisis will eventually subside. At best, a cure will come, or at least a vaccine. At worst, AIDS will burn its way through broad swaths of humanity, and then die down to the level of a pervasive endemic disease like malaria. Epidemics, like everything else in life, rise and fall; it is their nature.

And then?

I need to begin to imagine such a day—in my own life, in the life of the rest of the world. What will it mean when the end of the crisis really arrives? How will we think back on these years, and what will be our priorities then?

LOOKING BACKWARD

Much of this book has looked to the past, attempting to make sense of the past two decades by looking into the annals of human experience over most of a millennium. This is a risky exercise. The past, McGill University historian Nancy Partner warns, "incorrigibly slips into fiction"; she further cautions that history is "the definitive human audacity imposed on formless time and meaningless event."[1] Human beings, in other words, cannot simply *find* a meaning in the past, since there is no meaning there; instead, we must make it up for ourselves as we go along. This enterprise is perilous, but necessary. We must constantly join the present moment to memories of past experience, breaking and reassembling the pieces, seeking to find patterns in jumbled facts, and, to the best of our ability, make a picture of the world that we can understand.

We value history because, whatever its distortions and inaccuracies, it is a way of understanding and giving value to our collective human experience and collective human memory. As Oxford author and theologian C. S. Lewis (1898–1963) observed, "Humanity does not pass through stages as a train passes through stations; being alive it has the privilege of always moving yet never leaving anything behind."[2] Today is inseparable from yesterday and the days before, however subjectively we may understand them.

As this book has shown, one of the things humanity has not left behind is the interwoven association of sex with disease and sin. By looking at this complex web, we can learn a tremendous amount about what people have thought, believed, and seen as most crucial in their lives.[3] The records I have explored in this book are full of examples of suffering, courage, bravery, and compassion. They also abound in examples of people who have felt that they had a right, as the seventeenth-century English author L. S. wrote in his treatise on syphilis, to feel contempt for "others who have more of passion and less of prudence than themselves."[4] In some ways, seventeenth-century moralists and their modern counterparts are no different from the second-century Christians who believed that celibacy was the only path to salvation, and of whom St. Clement of Alexandria observed that "they set their hopes on their private parts." By condemning sex so vehemently, they make it far more important than it ought to be. Far better, I think, to see sex as a normal human function like eating and drinking, much as classical medicine did, and to deal with problems when they arise. To condemn people to suffer for their sexual behavior is irrational, immoral, and inhumane.

LOOKING INWARD

Social institutions and structures of belief exercise a tremendous influence over the ways in which people stay healthy or fall sick. "Diseases rarely 'just happen,'" argues AIDS ethicist Timothy Murphy. "More often than not, society's economic structure and moral values permit them to happen, make them inevitable."[5] When people have enough to eat and a clean environment, when they have good access to medical knowledge and care, and when they live in a society that values health highly, they are far less likely to suffer from chronic and epidemic diseases than when they do not. As French chemist and microbiologist Louis Pasteur (1822–1895) observed, whether diseases affect us depends less on the microbes we encounter than on how healthy we are to begin with.

People have long argued about whether individuals or social institutions bear the largest responsibility for disease. In the case I know the best, that of AIDS, both carry the burden. The ultimate responsibility for disease prevention falls on the individual, since he or she is the person who will have to bear the consequences when prevention fails. It is true that, in the face of infectious disease, many people are exceptionally careless with their lives and those of others, and I think such carelessness is deeply wrong. Nevertheless, I also believe that the institutions under whose auspices we organize and carry out our inner and outer lives—especially religious institutions and government—bear a great deal of responsibility as well, and in many cases, past and present, I believe they too have fallen short, and at great cost. Part of the reason for this failure, as I have argued in the preceding chapters, is that powerful people have felt free to view disease as an agent of God's wrath that punishes sexual behavior considered immoral, and hence to blame the sick for their own sufferings.

This kind of thinking to me seems appallingly presumptuous: who can know the mind of God? More intimately, it also reveals a failure of two qualities I believe are essential to civilized life, namely, charity and compassion. Without these, I believe, people and institutions lose the right to be considered reverent or just, and thus the right to claim moral authority.

Religion is a constant theme in this book, and the religion about which I have written the most is Christianity. There are historical and objective reasons for this choice: beginning at least in the early fourth century, when Constantine joined the Church and brought the Roman Empire into the fold along with him, Christianity has been by far the most powerful and influential religion in the West. But just as important as this historical fact has been my personal experience. Like many other American Jews, I was brought up with some knowledge of and regard for Jewish traditions, but also a strong awareness that I was a member of a minority religion in a country in which tolerance for minorities is widespread but sometimes dangerously thin. For generations my family has sought a role in the culture around us, and to a degree that seeking has distanced us from traditional Jewish life. Thus, some seventy years ago, my paternal grandfather changed his name from Jacob Abramowitz to Jack Allen. Had he not made that choice, had I gone through life more easily identifiable as a Jew, I suspect my experiences might have been quite different. As it is, I have had to make more of an effort to choose a Jewish identity, and have lived within Christian America without quite being of it.

Not one of my three siblings has married someone from a Jewish background, and I am sure that this pattern was working when I fell in love with Stewart Telfer. It has also affected my relationship with American culture in general, as I am attracted to, but also troubled by, values that I sometimes neither like nor understand. Part of the reason I needed to write this book was to come to terms with Christianity, not just for Stewart but also for myself.

What I have learned is that Christianity is not a monolith but a collection of many diverse strands of tradition and faith. It does contain elements of intolerance, and these are the parts of Christian belief I find it difficult to accept—particularly when they spill out beyond church walls, and when religious leaders claim the right to tell non-Christians how to think and act. I feel that doing so indicates a lack of respect for other people and for the aspects of the divine that they embody and enact in their lives. But I have also discovered and come to admire elements of Christianity that serve as an inspiration to me, including the exceptional value it accords to compassion for the suffering, caring for the unfortunate, and manifesting steadfast love for humanity in the face of the dire challenges life can provide. Having learned to see and admire these qualities, I can see better why Christianity has appealed to so many people for so long. Ultimately, I now know, it is intolerance and self-righteousness that I cannot respect, and these are unfortunately to be found in people of every faith, as well as in those of no faith at all.

These issues are directly tied, of course, to the matter of this book, which has looked at how people's morality has influenced their response to disease. This is of particular importance in the United States, a nation that is both exceptionally devout and extraordinarily diverse. As University of Chicago Divinity School professor Martin Marty has observed, "the American founding ideal is revolutionary: that all are equal simply by being human; that competing interests, even if based on ethnic, racial, or religious identities, must compete within this foundational political-philosophical framework."[6] America is a complex and profoundly pluralistic nation, and this identity cannot be reconciled with the dominance of any single view of religion, sexual morality, or health.

LOOKING FORWARD

The *pax antibiotica* of the 1960s and 1970s was at best a truce, and more probably an illusion. Over the past several decades, the globe has been bombarded with new infectious diseases, from Legionnaires' Disease and hantavirus to Ebola, Lassa, and Marburg fever.[7] Less spectacular but more threatening are the increasingly drug-resistant strains of routine infections like staphylococcus, gonorrhea, and TB. Far more common than the exotic newcomers, these are the diseases that are perilously close to overcoming all the defenses of the American and European health care systems today.[8]

As we face a virulent future, we have a tremendous amount to learn from the history of disease, as Yale historian John Boswell pointed out before he died from AIDS in 1994. "Meanness and cruelty, compassion and heroism seem to be reinvented in the face of each new disaster. It remains to be seen whether American society will learn more than earlier societies did, whether it can pass to posterity the wisdom it acquires, and how it will acquit itself morally during this time of trial."[9] The United States has handled some parts of this trial better than could have been expected, and some worse. I am deeply grateful for the lives that have been spared—including my own—and for disasters averted. Yet I still believe that the losses have been too great, and I believe that we incurred many of them because we, as a nation, failed to advance the cause of AIDS prevention as aggressively as we could and should have.

The flow of time cannot be reversed: what is gone is gone. But in a Greek myth I remember reading in my childhood, even the box of human trials and sorrows set loose by Pandora contained, under everything else, the small, redeeming treasure of hope. I do believe that there are ways to make the future better than the past—ways that are profoundly rooted in the greatest traditions of this nation. Author and journalist Dennis Altman noted that "one of the central questions raised by AIDS is the ability of the state to care for what both Hobbes and Jefferson saw as the first requirement of government, namely the protection of life itself."[10] Protecting the population against disease is a fundamental obligation of the government, and I have come increasingly to hold, as the United Nations has been asserting for some time, that health is a human right that must be recognized and upheld, even though at times it may chafe against individual notions of religious morality, civil liberties, and economic freedom.[11] If the people and institutions of this country focused their energies on enforcing this principle, rather than on sacrificing individuals' well-being to parochial views and partisan prejudices, the country as a whole would grow, not only in health and economic strength, but also in faith and righteousness.

All of us, individually and collectively, carry with us the losses and sufferings of our prior experience. I know that, at least for me, these will always color my life: people I loved are gone, and all the newfound friends and newborn children in the world can never replace them. But I have had the extraordinary fortune to survive this most recent plague, and I hope that a part of what I have learned to value in life, and of what I have learned in writing this book, will become something I can give to others. Like the past, loss is irreversible, but it is not vain as long as we can give it meaning. If I can help to increase courtesy, charity, and compassion in the world by writing about people I have known and people who died centuries before I was born, if I can increase understanding by writing about intolerance, then I believe that I will have done what was given me to do: to take the abundant kindness and love that have come my way and use them to help myself and others carry out the Jewish—and human—moral obligation of *tikkun olam,* healing a broken world.

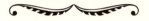

NOTES

INTRODUCTION

1. Lawrence K. Altman, "At AIDS Conference, a Call to Arms against 'Runaway Epidemic,'" *New York Times,* 29 June 1998.

2. For these and other statistics, consult <http://www.cdc.gov/nchstp/hiv_aids/stats.htm> and <http://www.thebody.com/sitemap.html>.

3. James Fletcher, M.D., "Homosexuality: Kick and Kickback?" *Southern Medical Journal* 77. 2 (February 1984): 149–50, citing Romans 1:26–27.

4. Pat Califia, "Tainted Love: Donna Minkowitz Is Reborn—and Reviled—by the Christian Right" (review of Minkowitz, *Ferocious Romance* [New York: Free Press, 1998], *POZ* (February 1999), available at <http://www.thebody.com/poz/culture/2-99/readthis.html>; Crimp, *AIDS: Cultural Analysis/Cultural Activism* (Cambridge: MIT Press, 1988), 8.

5. Carol Levine, Ph.D., MacArthur fellow and medical ethicist: interview, July 1996.

6. Marie de Maupeou Fouquet, *Recueil de rèmedes faciles et domestiques, choisis, experimentez & tres-approuvés, pour toute sorte de maladies, internes & externes, inveterées & difficiles à guerir. Recueillis par les ordres charitables d'une illustre & pieuse Dame, pour soulager les pauvres malades* (Dijon: Ressayre, 1678).

7. Harvey, *Great Venus,* 133; Quétel, *History,* 61; J. Worth Estes, *Dictionary of Protopharmacology: Therapeutic Practices, 1700–1850* (Canton, Mass.: Science History Publications, 1990), s.v. "hydrargus."

8. Thomas Vincent, *God's Terrible Voice in the City of London* (Cambridge: Samuel Green, 1667), 87.

CHAPTER ONE

1. *The Annals of Roger de Hoveden, Containing the History of England and of Other Countries of Europe from* A.D. *732 to* A.D. *1201,* 2 vols., trans. Henry T. Riley (London: H. G. Bohn, 1853; reprint, New York: AMS Press, 1968), 1: 204.

2. See O. J. Blum, "Thomas of York," *New Catholic Encyclopedia* (New York: McGraw-Hill,

1967–), 125; "Thomas (d. 1114), Archbishop of York," *Dictionary of National Biography,* ed. Leslie Stephen (New York: Macmillan and Co., 1886), 64: 3–5.

3. Nancy G. Siraisi, *Medieval and Early Renaissance Medicine: An Introduction to Knowledge and Practice* (Chicago: University of Chicago Press, 1990), 101–2.

4. See Aristotle, *On The Generation of Animals,* trans. A. L. Peck (Cambridge: Harvard University Press, 1963), 1.19, 726b; see also Julia Epstein, *Altered Conditions: Disease, Medicine, and Storytelling* (New York: Routledge, 1994), 146–51, 242 n. 68.

5. See generally Michel Foucault, *The History of Sexuality,* trans. Robert Hurley (New York: Vintage Books, 1985); David Halperin, *One Hundred Years of Homosexuality, and Other Essays on Greek Love* (New York: Routledge, 1989); Halperin, John J. Winkler, and Froma Zeitlin, eds., *Before Sexuality: The Construction of Erotic Experience in the Ancient Greek World* (Princeton: Princeton University Press, 1990); Kenneth Dover, *Greek Homosexuality* (Cambridge: Harvard University Press, 1978).

6. Madelain Farah, ed. and trans., *Marriage and Sexuality in Islam: A Translation of Al-Ghazālī's Book on the Etiquette of Marriage from the Ihyā'.* (Salt Lake City: University of Utah Press, 1984), 11–2, 31, 48–9, 60–4, 116; A. Bellamy, "Sex and Society," in *Society and the Sexes in Medieval Islam,* ed. Afaf Lufti al-Sayyid-Marsot (Malibu, Calif.: Undena, 1979), 30; Noel J. Coulson, "Regulation of Sexual Behavior under Traditional Islamic Law," in al-Sayyid-Marsot, ed., *Society and the Sexes,* 67–8; S. D. Goitein, "The Sexual Mores of the Common People," in al-Sayyid-Marsot, ed., *Society and the Sexes,* 47; Bürgel, "Love, Lust, and Longing: Eroticism in Early Islam as Reflected in Literary Sources," in al-Sayyid-Marsot, ed., *Society and the Sexes,* 92–3.

7. Vivian Nutton, "From Galen to Alexander: Aspects of Medicine and Medical Practice in Late Antiquity," in *Symposium on Byzantine Medicine,* ed. John Scarborough, Dumbarton Oaks Papers, 38 (Washington, D.C.: Dumbarton Oaks, 1983), 5.

8. Darrel Amundsen and Gary Ferngren, "The Early Christian Tradition," in *Caring and Curing: Health and Medicine in the Western Religious Traditions,* ed. Ronald L. Numbers and Darrel W. Amundsen (New York: Macmillan, 1986), 44–5, 53; Nutton, "From Galen to Alexander," 7–8.

9. Peter Brown, *The Body and Society: Men, Women, and Sexual Renunciation in Early Christianity* (New York: Columbia University Press, 1988), 134–5, 256, 294–5, with reference to Clement of Alexandria, *Stromateis;* Frank Bottomley, *Attitudes to the Body in Western Christendom* (London: Lepus Books, 1979), 6, 71.

10. Galen, "De locis affectis," 6.5, translated in Peter Brown, *The Body and Society,* 20.

11. See Danielle Jacquart and Françoise Micheau, *La médecine arabe et l'Occident médiéval* (Paris: Maisonneuve et Larose, 1990), 79.

12. Massimo Ciavolella, *La "malattia d'amore" dall'antichità al medioevo* (Rome: Bulzoni, 1976), 58–60.

13. See Jacquart and Claude Thomasset, *Sexuality and Medicine in the Middle Ages,* trans. Matthew Adamson (Princeton: Princeton University Press, 1988), 123.

14. Mary Frances Wack, *Lovesickness in the Middle Ages: The* Viaticum *and Its Commentaries* (Philadelphia: University of Pennsylvania Press, 1990), 32–4.

15. Bernard of Clairvaux, Letter 388, cited in Siraisi, *Medieval and Early Renaissance Medicine,* 14.

16. Cited in Darrel Amundsen, "The Medieval Catholic Tradition," in *Caring and Curing: Health and Medicine in the Western Religious Traditions,* ed. Ronald L. Numbers and Darrel W. Amundsen (New York: Macmillan, 1986), 91.

17. Ibid., 98.

18. See E. Ruth Harvey, *The Inward Wits: Psychological Theory in the Middle Ages and the Renaissance* (London: Warburg Institute, University of London, 1975), 20; also Rhazes, *Al-Hawi Fi'l-Tibb (Liber continentis in medicina)* (Brescia: Jacobus Britannicus, 1486); William of Saliceto, "Cyrurgia," in *Summa conservationis et curationis Gulielmi Placentini* (Venice: Bonetus Locatellus for Octavianus Scotus, 1502); Hildegard von Bingen, *Causae et curae,* ed. P. Kaiser, Biblioteca scriptorum graecorum et romanorum teubneriana, 133 (Leipzig: Teubner, 1903); and Aretaeus of

Cappadocia, *The Extant Works,* ed. and trans. Francis Adams, Sydenham Society 38 (London: Sydenham Society, 1856).

19. Arnald of Villanova, *Breviarium practice,* in his *Opera* (Lyons: F. Fradin, 1504) chap. 26, fol. 204r.

20. Kathleen McKernan, "Huntington Man Gets 4 Years; Defendant Tells Court He Performed Surgeries in Order to Help People," *Indianapolis Star,* 13 April 1999.

21. See Ralph Hexter, *Ovid and Medieval Schooling: Studies in Medieval School Commentaries on Ovid's* Ars amatoria, Epistulae ex Ponto, *and* Epistulae heroidum (Munich: Arbeo-Gesellschaft, 1986); and Peter L. Allen, *The Art of Love: Amatory Fiction from Ovid to the* Romance of the Rose (Philadelphia: University of Pennsylvania Press, 1992).

22. Bernard de Gordon, *Lilium medicinae* (Lyons: G. Rouillium, 1550), 210f. Similar advice is found in Avicenna's *Canon,* trans. Gerardus Cremonensis (Venis: O. Scotus, 1505).

23. See Jean de Saint-Amand, *Concordanciae,* ed. Julius Leopold Pagel (Berlin: G. Reimer, 1894), 2.7.114; compare Jacquart and Thomasset, 75, 115.

24. Gerard de Solo, commentary on book 9 of Rhazes's *Liber ad regem Almansorem* and unpublished *Determinatio de amore hereos,* cited in Wack, "The Measure of Pleasure: Peter of Spain on Men, Women, and Lovesickness," *Viator* 17 (1986): 191.

25. Plato, *Timaeus,* 91c, quoted in Ilza Veith, *Hysteria: The History of a Disease* (Chicago: University of Chicago Press, 1965), 7.

26. *Galen on the Affected Parts,* trans. Rudolph E. Siegel (Munich: S. Karger, 1976), bk. 6, p. 184 (Kühn, 417); see also bk. 4, pp. 182–3.

27. William of Saliceto, *Summa,* chap. 170, fols. 632v–634; see also chaps. 163 and 169. Trotula, Bernard, Peter of Spain, and Arnald made similar declarations: see Trotula of Salerno (Trocta salernitana), *De mulierum passionibus,* ed. Clodomiro Mancini, Scientia veterum, collana di studi della cattedra di storia della medicina dell'Università di Genova 31 (Genova: Università di Genova, 1962); Bernard de Gordon, *Lilium medicinae* (Lyons: G. Rouillium, 1550); Peter of Spain (Petrus Hispanus, later Pope John XXI), *Thesaurus pauperum* (Treasure chest of the poor), in *Practica Jo. Serapionis* (Lyons: Jacob Myt, 1525), fols. 253–72.

28. Arnald, *De regimine sanitatis salernitana,* in *Opera,* chap. 10; *Speculum medicine,* in *Opera,* chap. 83, fol. 132; *De regimine sanitatis regis aragonie,* chap. 6, in *Opera,* n.p.; *Tractatus de amore heroico,* in *Opera omnia,* ed. L. Garcia, Seminarium historiae medicae granatensis [et barchinone] 3 (Granada, 1985), chap. 4.

29. Arnald, *Breviarium practice,* chap. 9, fol. 222v.

30. Cited in John T. McNeill and Helena M. Gamer, *Medieval Handbooks of Penance* (New York: Columbia University Press, 1938), 168.

31. William of Auvergne (Guillaume d'Auvergne, Guilielmus Alvernus) *De sacramento matrimonii,* in *Opera omnia* (Paris: L. Billaine, 1674), chap. 9, 1.526; chap. 2, 1.513–4; Bartholomew, *Penitentiale,* 69, cited in James A. Brundage, *Law, Sex, and Christian Society in Medieval Europe* (Chicago: University of Chicago Press, 1987), 305; William of Auxerre (Guillaume d'Auxerre, Guilielmus Altissiodorensis), *Summa aurea* (Paris: N. Vaultier and D. Gerlier, 1500), bk. 2, tr. 17, chap. 4, fol. 73v; see also bk. 4, fol. 287r-v.

32. See Siraisi, *Medieval and Early Renaissance Medicine,* 44; Amundsen, "Medieval Catholic Tradition," 87, 92; and Jacquart and Thomasset, *Sexuality and Medicine,* 196.

33. Brundage, *Law, Sex,* 206, 247.

34. Ibid., 315.

35. St. Birgitta of Sweden, *Revelationes* 7.10, cited in Brundage, *Law, Sex,* 538.

36. William of Auxerre, *Summa aurea,* bk. 4, fol. 300v.

37. See William of Auvergne, *De anima,* pt. 33, in *Opera omnia,* 2.192; Vincent of Beauvais (Vincent de Beauvais, Vincentius Bellovacensis), *Speculum quadruplex sive speculum maius* (Graz: Akademische Druck- u. Verlagsanstalt, 1965), vol. 2, bk. 14, chap. 59, col. 1319.

38. *Dialogues of St. Gregory,* trans. E. G. Gardner (London, 1911), 55, cited in Bottomley, *Attitudes to the Body,* 104.

39. See Amundsen, "Medieval Catholic Tradition," 75; and Brundage, *Law, Sex,* 25.

40. Jacques Ferrand, *A Treatise on Lovesickness,* ed. and trans. Donald A. Beecher and Massimo Ciavolella (Syracuse, N.Y.: Syracuse University Press, 1990).

CHAPTER TWO

1. D. H. Pennington, *Europe in the Seventeenth Century,* 2nd ed. (London: Longman, 1989), 55.

2. Ann G. Carmichael, "Leprosy," in *The Cambridge World History of Human Disease,* ed. Kenneth F. Kiple (Cambridge: Cambridge University Press, 1993), 836; Danielle Jacquart and Claude Thomasset, *Sexuality and Medicine in the Middle Ages,* trans. Matthew Adamson (Princeton: Princeton University Press, 1988), 183.

3. Carmichael, "Leprosy," 834; Henri Marcel Fay, *Histoire de la lèpre en France: Lépreux et cagots du Sud-Ouest* (Paris: Honoré Champion, 1910), 19–26.

4. Carmichael, "Leprosy," 838; Charles Arthur Mercier, *Leper Houses and Medieval Hospitals* (London: H. K. Lewis, 1915), 5; Katharine Park, "Medicine and Society in Medieval Europe, 500–1500," in *Medicine in Society: Historical Essays,* ed. Andrew Wear (New York: Cambridge University Press, 1992), 72.

5. Fay, *Histoire,* 131; Stephen R. Ell, "Blood and Sexuality in Medieval Leprosy," *Janus* 7 (1984): 153; Mercier, *Leper,* 7; Albert Bourgeois, *Lépreux et maladreries du Pas-de-Calais (Xe–XVIIIe siècles)* (Arras: Commission départementale des monuments historiques du Pas-de-Calais, 1972), 66.

6. Peter Richards, *The Medieval Leper and His Northern Heirs* (Cambridge and Totowa, N.J.: D. S. Brewer and Rowman and Littlefield, 1977), 50, 36; James Young Simpson, "Antiquarian Notices of Leprosy and Leper Hospitals in Scotland and England," *Edinburgh Medical and Surgical Journal* 56 (1841): pt. 1, p. 311; Jean Imbert, *Les hôpitaux en France* (Paris: Presses Universitaires de France, 1958), 178.

7. Fay, *Histoire,* 113, 153, 178; Carmichael, "Leprosy," 839; Bourgeois, *Lépreux,* 66.

8. Timothy S. Miller, *The Birth of the Hospital in the Byzantine Empire* (Baltimore: Johns Hopkins University Press, 1985), 50–5, 86–7; Mercier, *Leper,* 2–4.

9. Miller, *Birth;* Michael Dols, "The Origins of the Islamic Hospital: Myth and Reality," *Bulletin of the History of Medicine* 61 (1987): 371–86.

10. Michel Mollat, "Les premiers hôpitaux (VIe–XIe siècles)," in *Histoire des hôpitaux en France,* ed. Jean Imbert (Toulouse: Privat, 1982), 25, 27; Mollat, "Floraison des fondations hospitalières, XIIe–XIIIe siècles," in Imbert, ed., *Histoire des hôpitaux,* 35; Natalie Zemon Davis, *Society and Culture in Early Modern France: Eight Essays* (Stanford: Stanford University Press, 1975), 49; Jacques Du Breul, *Le theatre des antiquitez de Paris, ou est traicté de la fondation des églises & chapelles de la cité, université, ville, & diocese de Paris* (Paris: Société des Imprimeurs, 1639), 1033.

11. Simpson, "Leprosy," pt. 2, pp. 399–400; Richards, *Medieval;* Mollat, "Floraison," 36–7.

12. Mollat, "Floraison," 36–7, 42; Richards, *Medieval,* v, 5, 131; Simpson, "Leprosy," pt. 1, pp. 319, 326–7; Jean Imbert, *Les hôpitaux en droit canonique* (Paris, 1947), 150.

13. See Miller, *Birth,* 5–6; Jean Pierre Gutton, "Mutations," in Imbert, ed., *Histoire des hôpitaux,* 157; Ernest Louis Coyecque, *L'Hôtel-Dieu de Paris au moyen âge: Histoire et documents* (Paris: H. Champion, 1889–1891); Katharine Park, *Doctors and Medicine in Early Renaissance Florence* (Princeton: Princeton University Press, 1985), 102.

14. Léon Le Grand, *Statuts d'Hôtels-Dieu et de léproseries: Recueil de textes du XIIe au XIVe siècle* (Paris: A. Picard, 1901), 178.

15. LeGrand, *Statuts,* 124, 133, 145, 151–64, 177; Michel Mollat, "La vie quotidienne dans les hôpitaux médiévaux," in Imbert, ed., *Histoire des hôpitaux,* 119–20; Jean-Pierre Gutton, "Hôtels-Dieu et hôpitaux de malades à l'âge classique (XVIIe–XVIIIe siècles)," in Imbert, ed., *Histoire des hôpitaux,* 205; Bronisław Geremek, *The Margins of Society in Late Medieval Paris,* trans. Jean Birrell (Cambridge: Cambridge University Press, 1987), 169; Imbert, *Les hôpitaux en droit*

canonique, 131; François Lebrun, *Se soigner autrefois: Médicins, saints, et sorciers aux 17e et 18e siècles* (Paris: Les Temps Actuels, 1983), 11–12; Katharine Park, personal communication.

16. Park, "Medicine," 71.

17. Bourgeois, *Lépreux*, 25, 26, 102.

18. LeGrand, *Statuts*, 224–5, 227; Mercier, *Leper*, 14.

19. Françoise Bériac, *Histoire des lépreux au moyen âge: Une société d'exclus* (Paris: Imago, 1988), 95, 115. Bériac is the primary source for material in this section.

20. Girolamo Fracastoro, *De contagione et contagiosis morbis et eorum curatione libri III*, trans. Wilmer C. Wright (New York: Putnam's Sons, 1930), sec. 213, p. 163; Fay, *Histoire*, 11; Jacquart and Thomasset, *Sexuality and Medicine*, 183–5; Andrew Nikiforuk, *The Fourth Horseman: A Short History of Epidemics, Plagues, Famine, and Other Scourges* (New York: M. Evans and Co., 1993), 31–2; Richards, *Medieval*, 62–3; Pierre Payer, *The Bridling of Desire: Views of Sex in the Later Middle Ages* (Toronto: University of Toronto Press, 1993), 109–10. Some studies have argued that, though leprosy is not sexually transmitted, there may be various clinical reasons why medieval physicians associated it with sex: see Simpson, "Leprosy," pt. 2, p. 124; Thomas Bateman, *A Practical Synopsis of Cutaneous Diseases* (London: Longman, 1813), 298; Richards, *Medieval*, xvi; Ynez Violé O'Neill, "Diseases of the Middle Ages," in *The Cambridge World History of Human Disease*, ed. Kenneth F. Kiple (Cambridge: Cambridge University Press, 1993); Ell, "Blood," 156–61.

21. LeGrand, *Statuts*, 184–5, 199–200, 227, 246–8; see also Mollat, "Floraison," 43; Richards, *Medieval*, 63.

22. Jean de Joinville, *Vie de St. Louis* (Paris, 1882), 10–11, cited in Bériac, *Histoire*, 105.

23. Mercier, *Leper*, 3–6; LeGrand, *Statuts*, xxvii n. 1, citing BN n. acq. lat. 608, p. 42 (1188 A.D.); and 3, citing Jacques de Vitry, *Historia occidentalis*, chap. 29; Richards, *Medieval*, 4, 71; Simpson, "Leprosy," pt. 1, p. .315; Nikiforuk, *Fourth Horseman*, 34.

24. Mercier, *Leper*, 11–2; Imbert, *Hôpitaux en droit*, 170–1.

25. Edicts of the diocese of Bayeux, from Imbert, *Hôpitaux en droit*, 171–3. See also Richards, *Medieval*, 123–4; Mercier, *Leper*, 11–3; Edouard Jeanselme, *Comment l'Europe, au moyen âge, se protégea contre la lèpre* (Brussels: Imprimerie médicale et scientifique, 1930), 143; Nikiforuk, *Fourth Horseman*, 26–7; Bourgeois, *Lépreux*, 54.

26. Mercier, *Leper*, 12.

27. Fay, *Histoire*, 113, 132, 153, 167, 169; Carmichael, "Leprosy," 839; Mercier, *Leper*, 8, 14–15; Geremek, *Margins*, 174; Simpson, "Leprosy," pt. 1, pp. 311, 323; pt. 2, pp. 412–3; Richards, *Medieval*, 36–50; Ell, "Blood," 153; Jeanselme, *Comment l'Europe*, 143; John Boswell, *Christianity, Homosexuality, and Social Tolerance: Gay People from the Beginning of the Christian Era to the Fourteenth Century* (Chicago: University of Chicago Press, 1980), 240–95 passim; cf. also David Nirenberg, *Communities of Violence: Persecution of Minorities in the Middle Ages* (Princeton, 1996).

28. Pierre Ruelle, ed., *Congés d'Arras* (Brussels, Paris: 1965); see also Paul Zumthor, *Histoire littéraire de la France médiévale* (Paris: Presses Universitaires de France, 1954).

29. Geremek, *Margins*, 16, 19, 52–3, 272.

30. Mollat, "Floraison," 46; Simpson, "Leprosy," pt. 2, p. 149; James Simpson, *Antiquarian Notices of Syphilis in Scotland in the Fifteenth and Sixteenth Centuries* (Edinburgh: Edmonston and Douglas, 1862), 22; Fay, *Histoire*, 183; Richards, *Medieval*, 86.

CHAPTER THREE

1. John Calvin, "Sermon 157, on Deuteronomy 28:25–29," in *Opera omnia quae supersunt* (Braunschweig, 1863–1900).

2. James Young Simpson, *Antiquarian Notices of Syphilis in Scotland in the Fifteenth and Sixteenth Centuries* (Edinburgh: Edmonston and Douglas, 1862), 4–6, 25.

3. Claude Quétel, *History of Syphilis*, trans. Judith Braddock and Brian Pike (Baltimore: Johns Hopkins University Press, 1990), 296 n. 69.

4. Charles Wickersheimer, "Sur la syphilis au XVe et XVIe siècles," *Humanisme et Renaissance*

4 (1936): 182–3; Michel Mollat, "Floraison des fondations hospitalières, XIIe–XIIIe siècles," in *Histoire des hôpitaux en France*, ed. Jean Imbert (Toulouse: Privat, 1982), 46; Simpson, "Antiquarian Notices of Leprosy and Leper Hospitals in Scotland and England," *Edinburgh Medical and Surgical Journal* 57 (1842): 149; and Simpson, *Syphilis*, 22.

5. J. Grünpeck, "Tractatus de pestilentiali scorra et hübscher Tractat von dem Ursprung des Bösen Franzos," in *The Earliest Printed Literature on Syphilis*, ed. Karl Sudhoff (Florence: R. Lier, 1924), 33; Ulrich von Hutten, *Of the Wood Called Guiacum, That Healeth the French Pockes*, trans. Thomas Paynel (London: Thomas Berthelet, 1540), 2v–3r; Gaspare Torrella, *Tractatus cum consiliis contra pudendagram seu morbum gallicum*, in Sudhoff, ed., *Earliest Printed Literature*, 190; Gideon Harvey, *Great Venus Unmasked: Or a More Exact Discovery of the Venereal Evil, or French Disease* (London: B. G. for Nath. Brook, 1672), 37; Conradinus Gilinus, "De morbo quem gallicum nuncupant," in Sudhoff, ed., *Earliest Printed Literature*, 254; Calvin, "Sermon 141 on Job 36," in *Sermons of Maister John Calvin, upon the Booke of Job*, trans. Arthur Golding (London: George Bishop, 1574; reprint, Edinburgh, Banner of Truth Trust, 1993); Darrel W. Amundsen, *Medicine, Society, and Faith in the Ancient and Medieval Worlds* (Baltimore: Johns Hopkins University Press, 1996), 313; Quétel, *History*, 41.

6. Harvey, *Great Venus; A New Method of Curing the French-Pox* (Amsterdam: For John Taylor and Thomas Newborough, 1690); see also Ernest Louis Coyecque, *L'Hôtel-Dieu de Paris au moyen âge* (Paris: H. Champion, 1889–1891), 104.

7. Nicolas Massa, "De morbo gallico liber," in *De morbo gallico omnia quae extant apvd omnes medicos cvivscvnqve nationis*, ed. Aloysius Luisinus (Venice: S. Zilettus, 1563); Girolamo Fallopius, *De morbo gallico liber absolutissimus* (Padua: Luca Bertellus, 1564), chap. 22; Harvey, *Great Venus*, 23; Richard Bunworth, *A New Discovery of the French Disease and Running of the Reins* (London: Henry Marsh, 1662), preface; Desiderius Erasmus, "Inns" and "A Marriage in Name Only," in *Colloquies of Erasmus*, ed. Craig Thompson (Chicago: University of Chicago Press, 1965).

8. Wickersheimer, "Sur la syphilis," 184ff.

9. Jacques Rossiaud, *Medieval Prostitution*, trans. Lydia G. Cochrane (Oxford: Basil Blackwell, 1988), 15, 18, 105; Natalie Zemon Davis, *Society and Culture in Early Modern France: Eight Essays* (Stanford: Stanford University Press, 1975), 69; H. G. Koenigsberger and George L. Mosse, *Europe in the Sixteenth Century* (London: Longmans, Green and Co., 1968), 65–8.

10. Rossiaud, *Medieval Prostitution*, 11–29, 31–3, 70, 130.

11. Augustine, *De ordine*, in *Aurelii Augustini, Contra academicos, De beata vita, necnon De ordine libri*, ed. William M. Green, Stromata patristica et mediaevalia (Utrecht: In Aedibus Spectrum, 1956), 2.4.12.

12. Rossiaud, *Medieval Prostitution*, 4–10, 22–3, 96; Bronisław Geremek, *The Margins of Society in Late Medieval Paris*, trans. Jean Birrell (Cambridge: Cambridge University Press, 1987), 214.

13. Rossiaud, *Medieval Prostitution*, 35, 130, 147, 158–9; André Biéler, *L'homme et la femme dans la morale Calviniste* (Geneva: Labor et Fides, 1963), 26, 108; F. G. Emmison, *Elizabethan Life: Morals and the Church Courts* (Chelmsford: Essex County Council, 1973), 2–32; James A. Brundage, *Law, Sex, and Christian Society in Medieval Europe* (Chicago: University of Chicago Press, 1987), 56–9.

14. Martin Luther, "A Sermon on the Estate of Marriage," in *Basic Theological Writings of Martin Luther*, ed. Timothy F. Lull (Minneapolis: Fortress Press, 1989), 631–2; Calvin, "Sermon 52 on Job 13"; Biéler, *L'homme et la femme*, 40, 133; Robert M. Kingdon, "Social Welfare in Calvin's Geneva," *American Historical Review* 76.1 (1971), 58.

15. For pro and con on this argument, see Emmison, *Elizabethan*, 2.32; Rossiaud, *Medieval Prostitution*, 50; Biéler, *L'homme et la femme*, 26.

16. Calvin, "Sermon 157."

17. Amundsen, *Medicine*, 328, 333, 347; Quétel, *History*, 19.

18. Fallopius, *De morbo*, 22r; Conradus Schellig, *In pustulas malas quem malum de Francia vulgus appellat consilium*, in Sudhoff, *Earliest Printed Literature*, 115.

19. L. S., *Prophylaktikon* (London, 1673), 51–2; Gilinus, "De morbo," 257; Quétel, *History*,

22, 58–9; Amundsen, *Medicine*, 348; Harvey, *Great Venus*, 64, 67, 107; Torrella, *Tractatus*, 201–6; Fallopius, *De morbo*, chap. 40; Johannes Widman (Meichinger), *Tractatus . . . de pustulis et morbo qui vulgato nomine mal de Franzos appellatur*, in Sudhoff, *Earliest Printed Literature*, 242; M. Dubé, *Le médecin et le chirurgien des pauvres*, 5th ed. (Paris: Couterot, 1678), vi; Alexis of Piedmont (Alexis Pedemontanus), *A Verye Excellent and Profitable Booke*, trans. Richard Androse (London: Henry Denham, 1569), 1.9, 1.20, 3.12–13; John Sadler, *Enchiridion medicum: An Enchiridion of the Art of Physick*, trans. R[obert] T[urner] (London: J. C. for R. Moone and Henry Fletcher, 1657), 13, 129.

20. Torrella, *Tractatus*, 202; Jean Liébault, *Thrésor des remedes secrets pour les maladies des femmes* (Paris: Jacques du Puys, 1587), 202–3; Erasmus, "A Marriage in Name Only," 409.

21. Alexis, *A Verye Excellent and Profitable Booke*, 2.44; Harvey, *Great Venus*, 110–1; François Lebrun, *Se soigner autrefois: Médecins, saints, et sorciers au 17e et 18e siècles* (Paris: Les Temps Actuels, 1983), 69–70; Quétel, *History*, 69–70, 84.

22. Robert H. Dreisbach and William O. Robertson, *Handbook of Poisoning*, 12th ed. (Norwalk, Conn.: Appleton and Lange, 1987), 238–43.

23. Harvey, *Great Venus*, 118–26; Quétel, *History*, 31; Von Hutten, *Of the Wood*, 6v; William Bullein, *The Book of Simples*, in *Bullein's Bulwarke of Defense against All Sicknesse* (London: Thomas Marsche, 1579), 7.74; Hieronymus Fracastorius, "De syphilide, seu morbo gallico lucubratio," in Luisinus, ed., *De morbo gallico*, bk. 3, chap. 10.

24. Ronald D. Mann, *Modern Drug Use: An Enquiry on Historical Principles* (Boston: MTP Press, 1984), 215; Quétel, *History*, 30, 65–6; G. R. Elton, *Reformation Europe* (New York: Harper and Row, 1963), 321; Harvey, *Great Venus*, 135–9; Sadler, *Enchiridion*, 41; Walter Pagel, *Paracelsus: An Introduction to Philosophical Medicine in the Era of the Renaissance* (New York: Karger, 1982), 24.

25. Mollat, "Dans la perspective de l'au-delà (XIVe–XVe siècles)," Imbert, ed., *Histoire des hôpitaux*, 70, 84–6, 95; Coyecque, *L'Hôtel-Dieu*, 178, 305, 310–1; Gutton, "Mutations," Imbert, ed., *Histoire des hôpitaux*, 141–2, 156; Henri Bordier and Léon Brièle, *Les archives hospitalières de Paris* (Paris: H. Champion, 1877), 88; Lebrun, *Se soigner*, 82–4.

26. Gutton, "Mutations," 143; E. M. Leonard, *The Early History of English Poor Relief* (London: Frank Cass and Co., 1965), 3, 11–16; Harold J. Grimm, "Luther's Contribution to Sixteenth-Century Organization of Poor Relief," *Archive for Reformation History* 61–2 (1970): 222–3.

27. Michael Dalton, *The Country Justice* (1635), cited in Leonard, *Early History*, 139–40.

28. Kingdon, "Social Welfare," 50, 67; Gutton, "Mutations," 145–6; Gutton, "L'enfermement à l'âge classique," Imbert, ed., *Histoire des hôpitaux*, 168, 174; Leonard, *Early History*, 25.

29. Keith Vivian Thomas, *Religion and the Decline of Magic* (London: Weidenfeld and Nicolson, 1971), 9, 14; Lebrun, *Se soigner*, 87.

30. Ann G. Carmichael, "Leprosy"; and Michael W. Dols, "Diseases of the Islamic World," both in *The Cambridge World History of Human Disease*, ed. Kenneth F. Kiple (Cambridge: Cambridge University Press, 1993), 838; and 336–8, 338–9. Japan, exceptionally, seems to have treated syphilis as an ordinary illness: Quétel, *History*, 651–2.

CHAPTER FOUR

1. Paul Slack, *The Impact of Plague on Tudor and Stuart England* (London: Routledge and Kegan Paul, 1985), 59.

2. Ann G. Carmichael, *Plague and the Poor in Renaissance Florence* (Cambridge: Cambridge University Press, 1986), 60.

3. Katharine Park, "Black Death," in *The Cambridge World History of Human Disease*, ed. Kenneth F. Kiple (Cambridge: Cambridge University Press, 1993), 613–4, see also Park, "Medicine and Society in Medieval Europe, 500–1500," in *Medicine in Society: Historical Essays*, ed. Andrew Wear (New York: Cambridge University Press, 1992); Slack, *Impact*, 30.

4. Cited in Slack, *Impact*, 239.

5. G. R. Elton, *Reformation Europe* (New York: Harper and Row, 1963), 294–5.

6. François Wendel, *Calvin: The Origins and Development of His Religious Thought*, trans. Philip

Mairet (New York: Harper and Row, 1963), 93–7; Elton, *Reformation*, 108; Calvin, Sermon 16 on Job 4 (72, col. B), referred to him as "that cursed creature that was burnt" because he said that the "Holy Ghost had not reigned as yet, but that he was to come"; *Sermons of Maister John Calvin, upon the Booke of Job*, trans. Arthur Golding (London: George Bishop, 1574; reprint, Edinburgh: Banner of Truth Trust, 1993).

7. Twenty years later, this book was held responsible for the collapse of ancient medicine "on the ground that it discredited the idea of the four humors and thus changed the method of curing diseases." Walter Pagel, *Paracelsus: An Introduction to Philosophical Medicine in the Era of the Renaissance* (New York: Karger, 1982), 1; Charles Webster, *The Great Instauration: Science, Medicine and Reform, 1626–1660* (New York: Holmes and Meier, 1975), xv; Guenter B. Risse, "History of Western Medicine from Hippocrates to Germ Theory," in Kiple, ed., *Cambridge World History*, 15; Richard Foster Jones, *Ancients and Moderns: A Study of the Rise of the Scientific Movement in Seventeenth-Century England* (St. Louis, Mo.: Washington University, 1961), 159, citing Thomas Willis, *Diatribæ duæ medico-philosophicæ*, 2nd ed. (London, 1660).

8. D. H. Pennington, *Europe in the Seventeenth Century*, 2nd ed. (New York: Longman, 1989), 168; Webster, *Great Instauration*, 349, 412. Webster notes (416) that a decimal currency for England was urged as early as 1641.

9. Of whom only the last were truly rejected by mainstream society: cf. Paul Dubé, *Le médecin et le chirurgien des pauvres* (Paris: Couterot, 1678), preface; François Lebrun, *Se soigner autrefois: Médecins, saints, et sorciers aux 17e et 18e siècles* (Paris: Les Temps Actuels, 1983), 38.

10. Margaret Pelling, "Healing the Sick Poor: Social Policy and Disability in Norwich 1550–1640," *Medical History* 29 (1985): 115–37.

11. See Lebrun, *Se soigner*, 52–6. Lebrun notes that the pulmonary circulation of the blood had been discovered by an Arab doctor in the thirteenth century, though this discovery, like that of Servetus, was ignored (55).

12. Cited in Jacques Rossiaud, *Medieval Prostitution* (Oxford: Basil Blackwell, 1988), 155; see also Carmichael, *Plague*, 123. Similarly, as Frank Wilson notes, a 1577 London sermon "pronounced this unconvincing syllogism: 'the cause of plagues is sinne, if you looke to it well; and the cause of sinne are playes: therefore the cause of plagues are playes,'" in *The Plague in Shakespeare's London* (Oxford: Clarendon Press, 1927), 51–2, citing both the Malone Society, *Collections*, 1.173 (ca. 1584); and T. Wilcocks, cited by Arber in his edition of Gosson's *The School of Abuse*, 8.

13. Michael W. Dols, *The Black Death in the Middle East* (Princeton: Princeton University Press, 1977), 89; Carlo M. Cipolla, *Public Health and the Medical Profession in the Renaissance* (Cambridge: Cambridge University Press, 1976), 60–1.

14. Carmichael, *Plague*, 17.

15. Pennington, *Europe*, 94; E. M. Leonard, *The Early History of English Poor Relief* (Cambridge: Cambridge University Press, 1900), 16.

16. Pennington, *Europe*, 28, 29, 55, 117; Slack, "Mortality Crises and Epidemic Disease in England, 1485–1610," in *Health, Medicine, and Mortality in the Sixteenth Century*, ed. Charles Webster (Cambridge: Cambridge University Press, 1979), 33; Bronisław Geremek, *The Margins of Society in Late Medieval Paris*, trans. Jean Birrell (Cambridge: Cambridge University Press, 1987), 176–7; Slack, "Mortality," 48.

17. Slack, *Impact*, 309.

18. Martin Luther, "Whether One May Flee from a Deadly Plague," in *Basic Theological Writings of Martin Luther*, ed. Timothy F. Lull (Minneapolis: Fortress Press, 1989), 737–50.

19. Laurent Joubert, *Erreurs populaires et propos vulgaires, touchant la médecine et le régime de santé* (Bordeaux: S. Millanges, 1579), title page, preface, 56–7.

20. Lebrun, *Se soigner*, 11–13, citing Claude Joly, bishop of Agen (1677) and Antoine Blanchard, a priest in the Vendôme (early eighteenth century).

21. H. G. Koenigsberger and George L. Mosse, *Europe in the Sixteenth Century* (London: Longmans, Green and Co., 1968), 87; Slack, *Impact*, 55; Ambroise Paré, *The Workes of That Famous Chirurgion Ambrose Parey*, trans. Tho. Johnson (London: Richard Cotes and William Du-

gard, 1649), bk. 22, chap. 2, pp. 535–6; Gideon Harvey, *The Family Physician, and the House Apothecary* (London: T. R[ookes]?, 1671), a2; Joubert, *Erreurs*, preface, 1–2, 55–7.

22. T[homas] V[incent], *God's Terrible Voice in the City of London* (Cambridge: Samuel Green, 1667), A2. The following pages contain numerous quotations from and paraphrases from this nineteen-page pamphlet.

23. Slack, *Impact*, 38.

24. I. D., *Salomon's Pest-House or Towre-Royall, Newly Re-Edified and Prepared to Preserve Londoners with Their Families, and Others from the Doubted Deluge of the Plague*, 2nd ed. (London: for Thomas Harper and Henry Holland, 1630), 1–2.

25. *London's Lamentation* (London: E. P. for John Wright Junior, 1641), 1–6.

26. John Donne, "The Litanie," *Divine Poems*, xxiii, in *Poems* (Oxford: Oxford University Press, 1912); cf. Keith Vivian Thomas, *Religion and the Decline of Magic: Studies in Popular Beliefs in Sixteenth- and Seventeenth-Century England* (London: Weidenfeld and Nicolson, 1971), 83.

27. Edward Lawrence, *Christ's Power over Bodily Diseases* (London: R. W. for Francis Tyton, 1662), 425.11.

28. Francis Herring, *Preservatives against the Plague* (London: for Thomas Pierrepont, 1665), 2; D., *Salomon's Pest-House*, 19, 20.

29. D., *Salomon's Pest-House.*

30. Karen Armstrong, *A History of God* (New York: Ballantine, 1993), 283.

31. Herring, *Preservatives*, epistle dedicatory, 2, p. 1; Lawrence, *Christ's Power*, 21, 32.

32. Lawrence, *Christ's Power*, 67, 71, 84–5, 98, 263; D., *Salomon's Pest-House*, 40.

33. Thomas Swadlin, *Sermons, Meditations, and Prayers; Upon the Plague* (London: Benson, 1637).

34. Swadlin, *Sermons*, 9–10, 15–6, 39–46, 86–7.

35. Slack, *Impact*, 35, 39; Thomas, *Religion*, 82, 85–6.

36. Slack, "Mortality," 49; and Slack, *Impact*, 34, 205, 288–91, 296, 309–10; Carmichael, *Plague*, 17, 90; Darrel W. Amundsen, *Medicine, Society, and Faith in the Ancient and Medieval Worlds* (Baltimore: Johns Hopkins University Press, 1996), 290; Wilson, *Plague*, 97.

37. Katharine Park, "Healing the Poor: Hospitals and Medical Assistance in Renaissance Florence," in *Medicine and Charity before the Welfare State*, ed. Jonathan Barry and Colin Jones (London: Routledge, 1991), 28.

38. Compare Thomas, *Religion*, 83.

39. Slack, for example, argues that the tendency to see disease as divine punishment is particularly Christian: *Impact*, 49.

CHAPTER FIVE

1. Dyan Elliott, "Pollution, Illusion, and Masculine Disarray: Nocturnal Emissions and the Sexuality of the Clergy," in *Constructing Medieval Sexuality*, ed. Karma Lochrie, Peggy McCracken, and James A. Schultz (Minneapolis: University of Minnesota Press, 1997).

2. Cited ibid., 7.

3. Jean Gerson, *De cognitione castitatis et pollutionibus diurnis, cum forma absolutionis* (Cologne: Ulrich Zel, 1470–1472); Gerson, *De confessione molliciei*, vol. 2 of *Opera* (Basel: Nicolaus Kesler, 1489), sec. 33.

4. Quoted in François Lebrun, "The Two Reformations: Communal Devotion and Personal Piety," in *Passions of the Renaissance*, ed. Roger Chartier, 96, vol. 3 of *A History of Private Life*, 5 vols., ed. Philippe Ariès and Georges Duby (Cambridge: Belknap/Harvard, 1989).

5. Aretaeus the Cappadocian, cited in E. F. Hirsch, "An Historical Survey of Gonorrhea," *Annals of Medical History* 2 (1930): 416.

6. Randolph Trumbach, "Sex, Gender, and Sexual Identity in Modern Culture: Male Sodomy and Female Prostitution in Enlightenment London," in *Forbidden History*, ed. John Fout (Chicago: University of Chicago Press, 1993), 90–98; Roy Porter, *English Society in the Eighteenth Century* (London: Penguin, 1990), 262–9.

7. Cited in Porter, *English*, 24.

8. Cited ibid., 177.

9. Philippe Ariès, *Centuries of Childhood: A Social History of Family Life*, trans. Robert Baldick (New York: Vintage, 1962), 100–2.

10. Cited in Dorothy Porter and Roy Porter, *Patient's Progress: The Dialectics of Doctoring in Eighteenth-Century England* (Cambridge: Cambridge University Press, 1989), 54.

11. William Buchan, *Domestic Medicine; or, The Family Physician* (Philadelphia: John Dunlap for R. Aitken, 1772).

12. Roger Chartier, "The Practical Impact of Writing," in *Passions of the Renaissance*, ed. Roger Chartier (Cambridge: Harvard/Belknap, 1989), 112–5; Porter, *English*, 167.

13. Voltaire, *Œuvres complètes*, vol. 42: *Dictionnaire philosophique*, article "Onan, Onanisme" (Paris, 1784), cited in E. H. Hare, "Masturbational Insanity: The History of an Idea," *Journal of Mental Science* 108 (1962): 20 n. 7a.

14. Hare, "Masturbational Insanity," 10.

15. Michelle Perrot, ed., *From the Fires of Revolution to the Great War*, trans. Arthur Goldhammer, 346, vol. 4 of *A History of Private Life*, ed. Philippe Ariès and Georges Duby (Cambridge: Harvard/Belknap, 1990).

16. Jacques Léonard, *La France médicale: Médecins et malades au XIXe siècle* (Paris: Gallimard, 1978), 178.

17. W. [Woodward, Samuel B.], "Remarks on Masturbation; Insanity Produced by Masturbation; Effections of Masturbation with Cases," *Boston Medical and Surgical Journal* 12 (1835). Emphasis in the original.

18. William Acton, *The Functions and Disorders of the Reproductive Organs*, 4th American ed. (Philadelphia: Lindsay and Blakison, 1875), 164; Perrot, *From the Fires*, 165.

19. Léonard, *La France médicale*, 243.

20. Baron Cuvier, *Discours à la Chambre des Pairs*, 1 May 1826; Barbey d'Aurevilly, "Pensée détachée no. 34," in *Works* (Pléiade edition), 2: 1628; both cited in Léonard, *La France médicale*, 243, 246.

21. Dr. J. Ch. Lebrun, *Des erreurs relatives à la santé* (Paris, 1824), 1; Dr. Léon Boyer, *Du rôle de la médicine et des médecins dans la société*, Congrès scientifique de France à Montpellier en décembre 1868 (Montpellier, 1869), both cited in Léonard, *La France médicale*, 204.

22. Ludmilla Jordanova, "The Popularisation of Medicine: Tissot on Onanism," *Textual Practice* 1 (1987).

23. Robert Latou Dickinson, "Bicycling for Women from the Standpoint of the Gynecologist," *American Journal of Obstetrics* 31 (1895).

24. T. de Bienville, *Nymphomania, or a Dissertation concerning the Furor Uterinus*, trans. Edward Wilmot (London: J. Brew, 1775).

25. Léopold Deslandes, *Manhood: The Causes of Its Premature Decline: With Directions for Its Perfect Restoration; Addressed to Those Suffering from the Destructive Effects of Excessive Indulgence, Solitary Habits, &c., &c., &c.*, translated from the French, with many additions, by an American Physician (Boston: Otis, Broaders and Co, 1843)

26. François Lallemand, *A Practical Treatise on the Causes, Symptoms, and Treatment of Spermatorrhea* (Philadelphia, 1858), 145, cited in Arthur N. Gilbert, "Doctor, Patient, and Onanist Diseases in the Nineteenth Century," *Journal of the History of Medicine and Allied Sciences* 30 (1975): 232–3; Lallemand, *Des pertes séminales involontaires*, 3 vols. (Paris: Béchet Jeune, 1836–1842).

27. Homer Bostwick, *A Treatise on the Nature and Treatment of Seminal Diseases* (New York: Burgess, Stringer and Co., 1847).

28. Everett Floyd, "An Appliance to Prevent Masturbation," *Medical Age* 6 (1888): 332–3, cited in Gail Pat Parsons, "Equal Treatment for All: American Medical Remedies for Male Sexual Problems 1850–1900," *Journal of the History of Medicine and Allied Sciences* 32.1 (1977): 63.

29. Samuel W. Gross, *A Practical Treatise on Impotence, Sterility, and Allied Disorders of the Male Sexual Organs*, 4th ed. (Philadelphia, 1890), preface, 44–5, cited in Parsons, "Equal," 67.

30. Louis Bauer, "Infibulation as Remedy for Epilepsy and Seminal Losses," *St. Louis Clinical Record* 6 (1879–1880).

31. Démétrius Alexandre Zambaco, "Onanisme avec troubles nerveux chez deux petites filles," *L'encéphale* 2 (1882).

32. Isaac Baker Brown, *On Surgical Diseases of Women*, 3rd ed. (London: R. Hardwicke, 1866); Brown, *On the Curability of Certain Forms of Insanity, Epilepsy, Catalepsy, and Hysteria in Females* (London, 1866).

33. Compare John Black, "Female Genital Mutilation: A Contemporary Issue, and a Victorian Obsession," *Journal of the Royal Society of Medicine* 90 (July 1997): 402–5.

34. J. H. Marshall, "Insanity Cured by Castration," *Medical and Surgical Reporter* 13 (1865): 363–4; R. D. Potts, "Castration for Masturbation, with Report of a Case," *Texas Medical Practitioner* 11 (1898): 8–9, both cited in H. Tristram Engelhardt, "The Disease of Masturbation: Values and the Concept of Disease," *Bulletin of the History of Medicine* 48 (1974): 244–5.

35. Cited in Parsons, "Equal," 63.

36. Quoted in Thomas Szasz, *The Manufacture of Madness* (New York: Harper and Row, 1970), 191.

37. Irving David Steinhardt, M.D., *Ten Sex Talks to Boys* (Philadelphia: J. B. Lippincott Co., 1914); Mary Wood-Allen, M.D., *Almost a Man*, 2nd ed. (Ann Arbor, Mich.: Wood-Allen Publishing Co., 1899).

38. Sir James Paget, *Clinical Lectures and Essays*, 2nd ed. (London, 1879), cited in Lesley A. Hall, "Forbidden by God, Despised by Men: Masturbation, Medical Warnings, Moral Panic, and Manhood in Great Britain, 1850–1950," in Fout, ed., *Forbidden History*, 295.

39. Freud, *Standard Edition* (London, 1971), 1: 180; 3: 150; cited in Engelhardt, "Disease," 241.

40. L. Emmett Holt, *Diseases of Infancy and Childhood* (New York: Appleton-Century, 1897), cited in René Spitz, "Authority and Masturbation: Some Remarks on a Bibliographical Investigation," *Yearbook of Psychoanalysis* 9 (1953): 126–7.

41. Baden-Powell, *Scouting* (London, 1908); and Baden-Powell, *Rovering for Success* (1922), cited in Robert H. MacDonald, "The Frightful Consequences of Onanism: Notes on the History of a Delusion," *Journal of the History of Ideas* 27 (1967): 430; Hall, "Forbidden," 301.

42. J. P. C. Griffith and A. G. Mitchell, *Diseases of Infants and Children*, 2nd ed. (1938), cited in Szasz, *Manufacture*, 200. See also Alfred C. Kinsey and Wardell B. Pomeroy, *Sexual Behavior in the Human Male* (Philadelphia: W. B. Saunders and Co., 1948), 513; and Szasz, *Manufacture*, 198, 201, citing Otto Fenichel, *The Psychoanalytic Theory of Neurosis* (New York: Norton, 1945).

43. Hall, "Forbidden."

44. G. Stanley Hall, *Adolescence: Its Psychology and Its Relations to Physiology, Anthropology, Sociology, Sex, Crime, Religion, and Education*, 2 vols. (New York: D. Appleton and Co., 1904), 1: 433–4; Vern L. Bullough, "The Development of Sexology in the U.S.A. in the Early Twentieth Century," in *Sexual Knowledge, Sexual Science: The History of Attitudes to Sexuality*, ed. Roy Porter and Mikulas Teich (Cambridge: Cambridge University Press, 1994), 313.

45. Compare *U.S. News and World Report*, 1 September 1986.

46. I am indebted to Rick Andrews, M.D., of the Department of Psychiatry of Cedars-Sinai Medical Center, Los Angeles, for these modern clinical diagnoses.

47. See Vernon A. Rosario, "Phantastical Pollutions: The Public Threat of Private Vice in France," in *Solitary Pleasures*, ed. Paula Bennett and Vernon A. Rosario (New York: Routledge, 1995); G. J. Barker-Benfield, *The Horrors of the Half-Known Life: Male Attitudes toward Women and Sexuality in America* (New York: Harper and Row, 1976), 165–6; Spitz, "Authority," 121.

CHAPTER SIX

1. Randy Shilts, *And the Band Played On: Politics, People, and the AIDS Epidemic* (New York: Penguin, 1988), 347, on the ABC show; Jerry Falwell, "AIDS: The Judgment of God," *Liberty*

Report (April 1987): 2; Albert R. Jonsen and Jeff Stryker, *The Social Impact of AIDS in the United States* (Washington, D.C.: National Academy Press, 1993), 131.

2. Gustav Niebuhr, "Week in Review: Kneeling at the Altar of Death: From Belief to Fanaticism," *New York Times,* 14 August 1995.

3. Mark Barnes, "Book Review: Toward Ghastly Death: The Censorship of AIDS Education," *Columbia Law Review* 89.698 (1989), 715, citing 133 *Congressional Record,* S 14204.

4. William C. Martin, *With God on Our Side: The Rise of the Religious Right in America* (New York: Broadway Books, 1996), 100.

5. Jonsen and Stryker, *Social Impact,* 131.

6. Reuter, "Buchanan: AIDS Is 'Retribution'," *New York Newsday,* 28 February 1992; Patrick J. Buchanan, "AIDS and Moral Bankruptcy," syndicated column, *New York Post,* 2 December 1987, 23.

7. *Congressional Record,* 14 October 1987, 514202–14220, cited in Douglas Crimp,"How to Have Promiscuity in an Epidemic," in *AIDS: Cultural Analysis/Cultural Activism* (Cambridge: MIT Press, 1988), 261; see also Jonsen and Stryker, *Social Impact,* 126.

8. Gina Kolata, "Congress, NIH, Open for AIDS," *Science* (29 July 1983): 436.

9. Shilts, *And the Band Played On,* 235.

10. Robert J. Blendon and Karen Donelan, "Discrimination against People with AIDS: The Public's Perspective," *New England Journal of Medicine* (13 October 1988): 1023–6.

11. Blendon and Donelan, "Public Opinion and AIDS: Lessons for the Second Decade," *Journal of the American Medical Association* 267.7 (19 February 1992), 983.

12. Barnes, "Toward Ghastly Death," 708–13, citing *New York Times,* 24 January 1987;133 *Congressional Record,* 20 October 1987, H 8801.

13. Charles Perrow and Mauro F. Guillen note, "The essentials of the disease—that it is a blood-borne virus infecting men and women, straights as well as gays, and that it is responsive to ridiculously cheap prevention measures (bleach and condoms) were all known in the first year, yet no education or warning campaign was mounted, nor was blood tested or the donors screened." *The AIDS Disaster: The Failure of Organizations in New York and the Nation* (New Haven: Yale University Press, 1990), 3.

14. Centers for Disease Control, *Basic Facts about Condoms and Their Use in Preventing HIV Infection and Other STDs* (Atlanta: Public Health Service/Centers for Disease Control, 1993, pamphlet; "Prevention May Cut AIDS Toll," *New York Daily News,* 8 August 1995; Editorial, "Some Hope on Third World AIDS," *New York Times,* 7 October 1996.

15. Pamela DeCarlo and Thomas Coates, *Does HIV Prevention Work?* (San Francisco: Center for AIDS Prevention Studies, 1995) fact sheet no. 1ER, <http://www.caps.ucsf.edu/preventionrev.html>.

16. Office of Technology Assessment, *How Effective Is AIDS Education?* Staff paper no. 3 (Washington, D.C.: Office of Technology Assessment, 1988), 56.

17. M. Rotheram-Borus, et al., "Reducing HIV Sexual Risk Behavior among Runaway Adolescents," *Journal of the American Medical Association* 266 (1991): 1237–41, cited in DeCarlo and Coates, *Does HIV Prevention Work?*

18. Jeff Stryker, "Prevention of HIV Infection: Looking Back, Looking Ahead," *Journal of the American Medical Association* 273.14 (12 April 1995): 1143–8.

19. Coates, Thomas, and Pamela DeCarlo, *We Know What Works in HIV Prevention—Why Aren't We Doing More of It?* (San Francisco: CAPS/Harvard AIDS Institute, 1996), fact sheet, citing D. Kirk et al., *Public Health Reports,* 109 (1994): 339–60; and S. M. Blower and A. R. McLean, *Science,* 265 (1994): 1451–4.

20. William C. Martin, *With God on Our Side: The Rise of the Religious Right in America* (New York: Broadway Books, 1996), 239.

21. James Warner, cited in Michael Fumento, *The Myth of Heterosexual AIDS: How a Tragedy Has Been Distorted by the Media and Partisan Politics* (Washington, D.C.: Regency Gateway, 1993), 193.

22. C. Everett Koop, *Koop: The Memoirs of America's Family Doctor* (New York: Random House, 1991), 220.

23. U.S. Congress, *AIDS Issues (Part I): Hearings before the Subcommittee on Health and the Environment of the Committee on Energy and Commerce,* House of Representatives, 101st Cong., 1st sess. (Washington, D.C.: Government Printing Office, 1984), 59; William Booth, "The Odyssey of a Brochure on AIDS," *Science* 237 (1987): 1410.

24. Martin, *With God,* 251.

25. William Bennett, *AIDS and the Education of Our Children: A Guide for Parents and Teachers* (Washington, D.C.: U.S. Department of Education, 1988), 4, 6.

26. Editorial, "What the Doctor Ordered," *Moody Monthly,* October 1988, 12.

27. Martin, *With God,* 250.

28. Saul Friedman, "Presidential Advice on AIDS Prevention," *New York Newsday,* 2 April 1987.

29. Koop, *Koop,* 208.

30. Peter Steinfels, "Southern Baptists Won't Give Out Surgeon General's Report on AIDS," *New York Times,* 23 September 1988.

31. Blendon and Donelan, "Discrimination," 1025; Koop, *Koop,* 224.

32. Interview, 6 March 1997.

33. *Congressional Record,* 14 October 1987, S 14202–7.

34. For this observation on safer-sex literature I am indebted to Temple University law professor Scott Burris.

35. Frank Van der Linden, "Disgusting Comic Book about AIDS," *Lebanon (Pa.) Daily News,* 25 October 1987; "Gay Comic," *Washington Times,* 8 October 1987; *Minneapolis Daily American,* 25 November 1987, 1–2.

36. James Kilpatrick, "Should Our Taxes Promote Safe Sodomy?" *Seattle Daily Times,* 19 December 1987.

37. Editorial, "More Gay-Bashing," *Nation,* 31 October 1987; for text see *Gay Men's Health Crisis et al. v. Dr. Louis Sullivan and James O. Mason* [hereafter *GMHC v. Sullivan*], United States District Court, Southern District of New York, 88 Civ. 7482 (SWK), 14 December 1989, 624 n. 4; Amendment to the Labor Health and Human Services for Fiscal Year 1988, P.H. no. 100–202.

38. 51 *Fed. Reg.* 3427 (1986), cited in Barnes, "Toward Ghastly Death," 714.

39. 42 U.S.C., Title 42, sec. 300ee(b), cited in *GMHC v. Sullivan,* 31 May 1991, 20.

40. *GMHC v. Sullivan,* 31 May 1991, 46–7; 26 June 1991, 20 n.16, 31; 11 May 1992, 294 n.32, 302, 303.

41. Harvey V. Fineberg, "Education to Prevent AIDS: Prospects and Obstacles," *Science* 239 (5 February 1988): 596; and John C. Cutler and R. C. Arnold, *American Journal of Public Health* 78 (1988): 372, cited in *GMHC v. Sullivan,* 26 June 1991, 4; "Study Supports Explicit AIDS Education," *San Jose (Calif.) Mercury-News,* 17 November 1987.

42. In *GMHC v. Sullivan,* 18 March 1991, 26.

43. Ibid., 11, 48–49; 26 June 1991, 1–2, 8–9.

44. Ibid., 11 May 1992, 278, 290, 291; 26 June 1991, 7 n. 4.

45. Richard L. Smith, *AIDS, Gays, and the American Catholic Church* (Cleveland, Ohio: Pilgrim Press, 1994), 27.

46. Arthur Heitzberg, "Catholics, Jews, and the Abortion Debate," *Reform Judaism* (Winter 1996): 87; Alan Correll, "Scientists Linked to the Vatican Call for Population Crisis," *New York Times,* 16 June 1994.

47. Ronald Modras, "Pope John Paul II's Theology of the Body," in *The Vatican and Homosexuality,* ed. Jeannine Gramick and Pat Furey (New York: Crossroad, 1988), 124, 120.

48. Josef Fuchs, *Natural Law: A Theological Investigation,* trans. Helmut Reckter and John A. Dowling (New York: Sheed and Ward, 1965), 141.

49. Cardinal Joseph Ratzinger, Congregation for the Doctrine of Faith, "Letter to the Bishops of the Catholic Church on the Pastoral Care of Homosexual Persons," in Gramick and Furey, ed., *The Vatican and Homosexuality.*

50. Ratzinger, "Letter," 5–6.

51. United States Catholic Conference Administrative Board, "The Many Faces of AIDS: A Gospel Response," *Origins* 17.28 (December 1987).

52. Ari L. Goldman, "U.S. Bishops Back Condom Education as a Move on AIDS," *New York Times,* 11 December 1987.

53. Bishop Anthony Bevilacqua, "The Questions Raised by School-Based Health Clinics," *Origins* 17 (3 September 1987): 189; U.S. Catholic Conference, "Many Faces," 489.

54. Smith, *AIDS,* 3, 65–59.

55. "Medical Science Is Not the Answer," notes a pamphlet published by the Medical Institute for Sexual Health (MISH): *The Facts about the STD Epidemic* (Austin, Tex.: Medical Institute for Sexual Health, 1996).

56. "Bishops to Order New AIDS Test," *Human Life International Reports* 6–8 (August 1988): 4, cited in Fumento, *Myth,* 169.

57. United States Department of Health and Human Services, PHS, CDC, *HIV/AIDS Surveillance Report* 9.2 (1999): 7–9, <http://www.cdc.gov/nchstp/hiv_aids/stats/hasr1002.pdf>.

58. *Marquis Who's Who* (Reed Elsevier Inc.), <http://web-lexis-nexis.com/universe/doc> accessed 3 May 1998; see also Kenneth L. Woodward, "Libels in the Cathedral," *Newsweek,* 1 April 1991, 59.

59. "Vatican AIDS Meeting Hears O'Connor Assail Condom Use," *New York Times,* 14 November 1989.

60. "O'Connor: Spiritual Focus Needed," *Newsday* [1987].

61. Linda Stevens, "Cardinal Is Top Speaker on AIDS," *New York Post,* 13 November 1989.

62. Linda Stevens and Rocco Parascandola, "Protests Rock St. Pat's: 111 Arrested in Protest Rally at Cathedral," *New York Post,* 11 December 1989.

63. Larry Celona and Dan Gentile, "Sunday Punch KOs St. Pat's," *New York Daily News,* 11 December 1989; Editorial, "Civil Disobedience vs. Uncivilized Behavior," *New York Daily News,* 12 December 1989; Editorial, "Sacrilege in St. Pat's," *New York Post,* 12 December 1989; Editorial, "The Storming of St. Pat's," *New York Times,* 12 December 1989; Maralyn Matlick, "Backlash-Wary Gays Rip Protest at St. Pat's," *New York Post,* 13 December 1989.

64. Linda Stevens and Richard Stein, "O'Connor Digs In," *New York Post,* 12 December 1989," *New York Daily News,* 12 December 1989.

65. Victoria Harden, Ph.D., NIH Historian, personal communication, July 1998.

66. Shari Roan, "When the Church and Medicine Clash," *Los Angeles Times,* 2 February 1995.

67. Isbell interview, 1995.

68. Peter Steinfels, "Catholic Bishops Vote to Retain Controversial Statement on AIDS," *New York Times,* 28 June 1988; Interview with Barbara R. Taylor, Ed.D., former coordinator of clinical and guidance services for Title I Services for the City of New York, 1996.

69. Bruce Lambert, "A Church-State Conflict Arises over AIDS Care," *New York Times,* 23 February 1990; Cindy Adams and Joe Nicholson, "O'Connor: City Urges Church to Teach Safe Sex," *New York Post,* October 1990.

70. Catherine Woodard, "Cuomo Defends Archdiocese on AIDS Care," *New York Newsday,* 10 January 1990; Thomas K. Duane, letter to Richard Yezzo, President, St. Claire's Hospital, 22 February 1994.

71. Interview with Professor Ron Bayer, Columbia University School of Public Health, November 1996; Barbara Taylor interview, 1997.

72. "The Bad News," *Time,* 2 December 1996, 25; "The Nation's Most Common Infections Are Sexual," *New York Times,* 20 October 1996; Joe S. McIlhaney, M.D., undated fundraising letter for MISH.

73. Josh McDonnell, "The Teen Sex Crisis," *Religious Broadcasting,* January 1987, 17, in C. Everett Koop Papers, National Library of Medicine.

74. Helen Schietinger, *Good Intentions: A Report on Federal HIV Prevention Programs* (Washington, D.C.: AIDS Action Council, 1991), Conclusions, 3.

75. Blendon and Donelan, "Public Opinion," 984.

76. Schietinger, *Good Intentions*, 20.

77. Guardian Family Association, advertisement, *New York Post*, 22 March 1993.

78. "School Parents Call Halt to Use of a Book on AIDS," *New York Times*, 14 March 1996.

79. Coates and DeCarlo, *We Know What Works*.

80. "Boston Cardinal: Skip AIDS Classes," *USA Today*, 22 May 1989; "Cardinal Assails AIDS Lesson for Boston Schools," *New York Times*, 22 May 1989.

81. Joe Nicholson, "Bishop Pulls Plug on State AIDS Book," *New York Post*, 19 September 1992.

82. B. D. Cohen, "Religious Double Standard," *New York Newsday*, 23 February 1993.

83. Sam Dillon, "Board Removes Fernandez as New York Schools Chief after Stormy 3-Year Term," *New York Times*, 11 February 1993.

84. Joseph Fernandez, with John Underwood, *Tales out of School: Joseph Fernandez's Crusade to Rescue American Education* (Boston: Little, Brown), 1993.

85. Joseph Berger, "Teaching about Gay Life Is Pressed by Chancellor," *New York Times* 17 November 1992; Steven Lee Myers, "Queens School Board Suspended in Fight on Gay-Life Curriculum," *New York Times*, 2 December 1992.

86. Dillon, "Board."

87. Anna Quindlen, "Public and Private: Church and State," *New York Times*, 17 February 1993.

88. Mireya Navarro, "Group Brings New AIDS Ads in Subways," *New York Times*, 14 January 1994; Ray Kerrison, "Sleazy AIDS Ads Take the Gay Train," *New York Post*, 19 January 1994; Editorial, "Porn Rides the Rails," *New York Post*, 20 January 1994.

89. Kristina Campbell, "Explicit AIDS Ads Riding NYC, Boston Trains," *Washington Blade*, 21 January 1994; Editorial, " 'Family Values' Won't Save Our Youth," *Our Town* (New York), 27 January 1994; Dan Janison, "Pols All Hot and Bothered by Subway AIDS Ads." *New York Post*, 28 January 1994; Jeff Richardson, Letter to the editor, *New York Post*, 29 January 1994; Editorial, "Little Ad-Vantage to This Campaign," *New York Daily News*, 30 January 1994; "Ignore Those Subway Ads," *Tablet* (Diocese of Brooklyn, New York), 5 February 1994; Jeff Richardson, Letter to the editor, *New York Daily News*, 14 February 1994.

90. Centers for Disease Control, "Condoms for Prevention of Sexually Transmitted Diseases," *Morbidity and Mortality Weekly Reports* 37.9 (11 March 1988): 134.

91. Blendon and Donelan, "Public Opinion," 982. See also Pamela DeCarlo, *Do Condoms Work?* (San Francisco: Center for AIDS Prevention Studies, UCSF/Harvard AIDS Institute, 1995), fact sheet.

92. Lawrence Goodman, "Catholic Group to Explode Condom Secret," *New York Post*, 27 April 1994; Jessie Mangaliman, "Ads on Two Tracks: Dueling Posters Put Views on Condoms into the Subways," *New York Newsday*, 18 May 1994; Editorial, "Follow the Facts: Condoms Work, Distortions Don't," *New York Newsday*, 18 May 1994; Mark Mooney, "Commish Slams Anti-Condom Ads," *New York Daily News*, 23 May 1994.

93. Interview with Dr. Theo Sandfort, Professor, University of Utrecht, Netherlands, summer 1995; Martin Foreman, Director of the Panos Institute's AIDS in the Americas program, interview, August 1994; "Ray of Hope in Uganda in War against HIV," *AIDS Weekly Plus*, 3 March 1997, 19ff.; D. Shepard, "The Cost of AIDS: Prevention and Education," *World Health* 50.5 (1997): 20ff.; "Changes in Thai Sexual Behavior Lower HIV Spread," *AIDS Weekly Plus*, 2 June 1997, 24ff. I am indebted to Michelle Ogawa for these references.

94. Gabriel Rotello, *Sexual Ecology: AIDS and the Destiny of Gay Men* (New York: Dutton, 1997), 138; cf. P. Cameron et al., "Sexual Orientation and Sexually Transmitted Disease," *Nebraska Medical Journal* 70 (1985): 292–5, for further statistics on the frequency of STD transmission among gay men.

95. Ronald J. Sider, "AIDS: An Evangelical Perspective," *Christian Century* 105.1 (6 January 1998) 11.

96. Jonsen and Stryker, *Social Impact*, 145, 148; Fumento, Myth, 191; Metropolitan Community Church, *AIDS: Is It God's Judgment?* (Los Angeles, n.d.), pamphlet; Ari L. Goldman, "Epis-

copal Bishop Criticizes Catholic Church," *New York Times,* 1 April 1993; Rabbi Joseph Edelheit, "AIDS: A Transformative Challenge for Clergy" (lecture, n.p., n.d.), 2, 7.

97. Francis, cited in Elinor Burkett, *The Gravest Show on Earth: America in the Age of AIDS* (New York: Picador, 1995), 292.

98. Jeff Stryker, "Broken Promises in the AIDS War," *San Francisco Examiner,* 4 August 1994; Stryker, "Onan the Barbarian," *San Francisco Examiner,* 1 January 1995; Rick Weiss, "President to Introduce National AIDS 'Strategy,'" *Valley News (White River Junction, Vt.; Lebanon, N.H.),* 17 December 1996.

99. *Ricky Ray Hemophilia Relief Fund Act of 1997,* 105th Cong., H.R. 1023, introduced into the House of Representatives on 11 March 1997, passed on 19 May and received in the Senate on 31 July 1998: Congressional Universe, Lexis-Nexis, <http://web.lexis-nexis.com/cis>, retrieved 28 August 1998.

100. Perrow and Guillen, *The AIDS Disaster,* 3; Office of Technology Assessment, *How Effective,* 56; interview with Sandfort; James G. Kahn and Pamela DeCarlo, *Is HIV Prevention a Good Investment?* (San Francisco: Center for AIDS Prevention Studies, UCSF/Harvard AIDS Institute, 1995.)

101. Smith, *AIDS,* xiii; Elizabeth Kübler-Ross, *AIDS: The Ultimate Challenge* (New York: Macmillan, 1987), 24, cited in Timothy F. Murphy, *Ethics in an Epidemic: AIDS, Morality, and Culture* (Berkeley: University of California Press, 1994), 4.

102. Interview with Carol Levine, MacArthur Fellow and director of the Orphan Project, New York, 1 July 1996.

CONCLUSION

1. Nancy Partner, "Making Up Lost Time: Writing on the Writing of History," *Speculum* 61.1 (January 1986): 97–8.

2. C. S. Lewis, *The Allegory of Love,* 2, cited in John M. Boswell, *Christianity, Homosexuality, and Social Tolerance* (Chicago: University of Chicago Press, 1980), 301.

3. On the revelatory value of medical history, see Claude Quétel, *History of Syphilis,* trans. Judith Braddock and Brian Pike (Baltimore: Johns Hopkins University Press, 1990), 2; Victoria A. Harden and Guenter B. Risse, *AIDS and the Historian* (Bethesda, Md.: National Institutes of Health, 1991), 7 (with reference to Charles Rosenberg, "What Is an Epidemic?" *Daedalus* 118 [1989]: 1–17); and Allan M. Brandt, "AIDS: From Social History to Social Policy," *Law, Medicine, and Health Care* 14.5–6 (December 1986): 231.

4. L. S., *Prophylaktikon* (London, 1673), 15.

5. Timothy F. Murphy, *Ethics in an Epidemic: AIDS, Morality, and Culture* (Berkeley: University of California Press, 1994), 170; see also Jonathan Mann, Daniel J. M. Tarantola, and Thomas W. Netter, eds., *AIDS in the World: A Global Report* (Cambridge: Harvard University Press, 1992), 19.

6. Martin Marty and R. Scott Appleby, *The Glory and the Power: The Fundamentalist Challenge to the Modern World* (Boston: Beacon Press, 1992), 193.

7. See, generally, Laurie Garrett, *The Coming Plague: Newly Emerging Diseases in a World out of Balance* (New York: Farrar, Straus and Giroux, 1994).

8. See ibid., with special reference to J. Lederberg, R. E. Shope, and S. C. Oaks, Jr., *Emerging Infections: Microbial Threats to Health in the United States,* Institute of Medicine Reports (Washington, D.C.: National Academy Press, 1992).

9. John Boswell, "Social History: Disease and Homosexuality," in *AIDS and Sex,* ed. Bruce Voeller, June Reinisch, and Michael Gottlieb, Kinsey Institute Series (New York: Oxford University Press, 1990), 181.

10. Dennis Altman, *AIDS in the Mind of America* (Garden City, N.Y.: Anchor Books, 1987), 26–7.

11. See, e.g., Jonathan Mann et al., eds., *AIDS in the World,* 347, 538.

BIBLIOGRAPHY

A New Method of Curing the French-Pox. Amsterdam: For John Taylor and Thomas Newborough, 1690.

Acton, William. *The Functions and Disorders of the Reproductive Organs in Youth, Adult Age, and Advanced Life, Considered in Their Physiological, Social, and Psychological Relations.* 4th American ed. Philadelphia: Lindsay and Blakiston, 1875.

Alexis of Piedmont (Alexis Pedemontanus). *A Verye Excellent and Profitable Booke Conteining Six Hundred Foure Score and Odde Experienced Medicines, Apperteyning unto Phisick and Surgerie.* . . . Translated by Richard Androse. London: Henry Denham, 1569.

Allen, Peter L. *The Art of Love: Amatory Fiction from Ovid to the* Romance of the Rose. Philadelphia: University of Pennsylvania Press, 1992.

Altman, Dennis. *AIDS in the Mind of America.* Garden City, N.Y.: Anchor Books, 1987.

Altman, Lawrence K. "At AIDS Conference, a Call to Arms against 'Runaway Epidemic.'" *New York Times,* 29 June 1998.

American Medical Association. *American Medical Directory: A Register of Legally Qualified Physicians of the United States.* 8th ed. Chicago: American Medical Association, 1923.

———. *American Medical Directory: A Register of Legally Qualified Physicians of the United States and Canada.* Chicago: American Medical Association, 1909.

American Psychiatric Association. *DSM-IV: Diagnostic and Statistical Manual of Mental Disorders.* 4th ed. Washington, D.C.: American Psychiatric Association, 1994.

Amundsen, Darrel W. *Medicine, Society, and Faith in the Ancient and Medieval Worlds.* Baltimore: Johns Hopkins University Press, 1996.

———. "The Medieval Catholic Tradition." In *Caring and Curing: Health and Medicine in the Western Religious Traditions,* ed. Ronald L. Numbers and Darrel W. Amundsen, 65–107. New York: Macmillan, 1986.

Amundsen, Darrel W., and Gary Ferngren. "The Early Christian Tradition." In *Caring and Curing: Health and Medicine in the Western Religious Traditions,* ed. Ronald L. Numbers and Darrel W. Amundsen, 40–64. New York: Macmillan, 1986.

Aretaeus of Cappadocia. *The Extant Works of Arataeus the Cappadocian.* Edited and translated by Francis Adams. Sydenham Society 38. London: Sydenham Society, 1856.

Ariès, Philippe. *Centuries of Childhood: A Social History of Family Life.* Translated by Robert Baldick. New York: Vintage, 1962.

Aristotle. *On the Generation of Animals.* Translated by A. L. Peck. Cambridge: Harvard University Press, 1963.

Armstrong, Karen. *A History of God.* New York: Ballantine, 1993.

Arnald of Villanova (Arnaldus de Villanova). *Breviarium practice.* In *Opera.* Lyons: F. Fradin, 1504.

————. *De regimine sanitatis regis Aragonie.* In *Opera.* Lyons: F. Fradin, 1504.

————. *De regimine sanitatis salernitana.* In *Opera.* Lyons: F. Fradin, 1504.

————. *Speculum medicine.* In *Opera.* Lyons: F. Fradin, 1504.

————. *Tractatus de amore heroico.* In *Opera omnia,* ed. L. Garcia. Seminarium historiae medicae granatensis, seminarium historiae medicae barchinone, vol. 3. Grenada, 1985.

Augustine. "De ordine." In *Aurelii Augustini, Contra academicos, De beata vita, necnon De ordine libri,* edited by William M. Green. Stromata patristica et mediaevalia. Utrecht: In Aedibus Spectrum, 1956.

Avicenna (Abū 'Ali Husayn ibn-'Abdullāh ibn Sīna). *Canon.* Translated by Gerardus Cremonensis. Venice: O. Scotus, 1505.

"The Bad News." *Time,* 2 December 1996.

Barker-Benfield, G. J. *The Horrors of the Half-Known Life: Male Attitudes toward Women and Sexuality in America.* New York: Harper and Row, 1976.

Barnes, Mark. "Book Review: Toward Ghastly Death: The Censorship of AIDS Education." *Columbia Law Review* 89 (1989): 698–724.

Bateman, Thomas. *A Practical Synopsis of Cutaneous Diseases.* London: Longman, 1813.

Bauer, Louis. "Infibulation as Remedy for Epilepsy and Seminal Losses." *St. Louis Clinical Record* 6 (1879–1880): 163–5.

Bell, Charles W. "'Over My Dead Body,' Angry O'Connor: Protesters Will Never Stop the Mass." *New York Daily News,* 12 December 1989.

Bellamy, A. "Sex and Society." In *Society and the Sexes in Medieval Islam,* ed. Afaf Lufti al-Sayyid-Marsot. Malibu, Calif.: Undena, 1979.

Bennett, William. *AIDS and the Education of Our Children: A Guide for Parents and Teachers.* Washington D.C.: U.S. Department of Education, 1988.

Berger, Joseph. "Teaching about Gay Life Is Pressed by Chancellor." *New York Times,* 17 November 1992.

Bériac, Françoise. *Histoire des lépreux au moyen âge: Une société d'exclus.* Paris: Imago, 1988.

Beverland, Adriaan. *De fornicatione cavenda admonitio; sive adhortatio ad pudicitiam et castitatem.* 2nd ed. London: C. Bateman, 1697.

Bevilacqua, Bishop Anthony. "The Questions Raised by School-Based Health Clinics." *Origins* 17 (3 September 1987): 187–9.

Biéler, André. *L'homme et la femme dans la morale calviniste: La doctrine réformée sur l'amour, le mariage, le célibat, le divorce, l'adultère, et la prostitution, considérée dans son cadre historique.* Geneva: Labor et Fides, 1963.

Bienville, T. de. *Nymphomania, or a Dissertation concerning the Furor Uterinus.* Translated by Edward Wilmot. London: J. Brew, 1775.

Black, John. "Female Genital Mutilation: A Contemporary Issue, and a Victorian Obsession." *Journal of the Royal Society of Medicine* 90 (July 1997): 402–5.

Blendon, Robert J., and Karen Donelan. "Discrimination against People with AIDS: The Public's Perspective." *New England Journal of Medicine* (13 October 1988): 1022–6.

————. "Public Opinion and AIDS: Lessons for the Second Decade." *Journal of the American Medical Association* 267.7 (19 February 1992): 981–6.

Booth, William. "The Odyssey of a Brochure on AIDS." *Science* 237 (1987): 1410.

Bordier, Henri, and Léon Brièle. *Les archives hospitalières de Paris.* Paris: H. Champion, 1877.

"Boston Cardinal: Skip AIDS Classes." *USA Today,* 22 May 1989.

Bostwick, Homer. *A Treatise on the Nature and Treatment of Seminal Diseases, Impotency, and Other*

Kindred Affections: With Practical Directions for the Management and Removal of the Cause Producing Them; Together with Hints to Young Men. New York: Burgess, Stringer and Co., 1847.

Boswell, John M. *Christianity, Homosexuality, and Social Tolerance: Gay People from the Beginning of the Christian Era to the Fourteenth Century.* Chicago: University of Chicago Press, 1980.

———. "Social History: Disease and Homosexuality." In *AIDS and Sex*, ed. Bruce Voeller, June Reinisch, and Michael Gottlieb. Kinsey Institute Series. New York: Oxford University Press, 1990.

Bottomley, Frank. *Attitudes to the Body in Western Christendom.* London: Lepus Books, 1979.

Bourgeois, Albert. *Lépreux et maladreries du Pas-de-Calais (Xe–XVIIIe siècles).* Arras: Commission départementale des monuments historiques du Pas-de-Calais, 1972.

Brandt, Allan M. "AIDS: From Social History to Social Policy." *Law, Medicine, and Health Care* 14.5–6 (December 1986): 231–42.

Brown, G. H. *Lives of the Fellows of the Royal College of Physicians of London, 1826–1925.* London: Royal College of Physicians, 1955.

Brown, Isaac Baker. *On the Curability of Certain Forms of Insanity, Epilepsy, Catalepsy, and Hysteria in Females.* London, 1866.

———. *On Surgical Diseases of Women.* 3rd ed. London: R. Hardwicke, 1866.

Brown, Peter Robert. *The Body and Society: Men, Women, and Sexual Renunciation in Early Christianity.* New York: Columbia University Press, 1988.

Brundage, James A. *Law, Sex, and Christian Society in Medieval Europe.* Chicago: University of Chicago Press, 1987.

Buchan, William, M.D. *Domestic Medicine; or, the Family Physician: Being an Attempt to Render the Medical Art More Generally Useful, by Shewing People What Is in Their Own Power Both with Respect to the Prevention and Cure of Diseases.* Philadelphia: John Dunlap for R. Aitken, 1772.

Buchanan, Patrick J. "AIDS and Moral Bankruptcy." *New York Post*, 2 December 1987.

Bullein, William. *The Book of Simples.* In *Bulleins Bulwarke of Defense against All Sicknesse, Soarenesse, and Woundes That Doe Dayly Assaulte Mankinde: Which Bulwarke Is Kept with Hilarius the Gardener, and Health the Physicion* . . . . London: Thomas Marsche, 1579.

Bullough, Vern A. "The Development of Sexology in the U.S.A. in the Early Twentieth Century." In *Sexual Knowledge, Sexual Science: The History of Attitudes to Sexuality*, ed. Roy Porter and Mikulas Teich, 303–22. Cambridge: Cambridge University Press, 1994.

Bunworth, Richard. *A New Discovery of the French Disease and Running of the Reins: Their Causes, Signs, with Plain and Easie Direction of Perfect Curing the Same.* London: Henry Marsh, 1662.

Bürgel, J. C. "Love, Lust, and Longing: Eroticism in Early Islam as Reflected in Literary Sources." In *Society and the Sexes in Medieval Islam*, ed. Afaf Lufti al-Sayyid-Marsot, 81–117. Malibu, Calif.: Undena, 1979.

Burkett, Elinor. *The Gravest Show on Earth: America in the Age of AIDS.* New York: Picador, 1995.

Butler, Samuel W. *The Medical Register and Directory of the United States.* Philadelphia: Office of the Medical and Surgical Reporter, 1874.

C., J. F. "Obituary: Isaac Baker Brown, F.R.C.S." *Medical Times and Gazette*, no. 1 (8 February 1873): 155–6.

Calvin, John. "Sermon 157, on Deuteronomy 28:25–29." In *Opera omnia quae supersunt*, 404. Braunschweig, 1863–1900.

———. *Sermons of Maister John Calvin, upon the Booke of Job.* Translated by Arthur Golding. London: George Bishop, 1574. Reprint, Edinburgh: Banner of Truth Trust, 1993.

Cameron, P., et al. "Sexual Orientation and Sexually Transmitted Disease." *Nebraska Medical Journal* 70 (1985): 292–9.

Campbell, Kristina. "Explicit AIDS Ads Riding NYC, Boston Trains." *Washington Blade*, 21 January 1994.

"Cardinal Assails AIDS Lesson for Boston Schools." *New York Times*, 22 May 1989.

Carmichael, Ann G. "Leprosy." In *The Cambridge World History of Human Disease*, ed. Kenneth F. Kiple, 834–9. Cambridge: Cambridge University Press, 1993.

———. *Plague and the Poor in Renaissance Florence*. Cambridge: Cambridge University Press, 1986.

Catholic League for Religious and Civil Rights. *Want to Know a Dirty Little Secret? Condoms Don't Save Lives*. Subway advertisement, New York City. Catholic League, 1994.

Catholic University of America. *New Catholic Encyclopedia*. New York: McGraw-Hill, 1967.

Celona, Larry, and Dan Gentile. "Sunday Punch KOs St. Pat's." *New York Daily News*, 11 December 1989.

Centers for Disease Control. *Basic Facts about Condoms and Their Use in Preventing HIV Infection and Other STDs*. Atlanta: Public Health Service/Centers for Disease Control and Prevention, 1993. Pamphlet. <http://www.thebody.com>

———. "Condoms for Prevention of Sexually Transmitted Diseases." *Morbidity and Mortality Weekly Reports* 37.9 (11 March 1988): 134ff.

———. "Pneumocystis Pneumonia—Los Angeles." *Morbidity and Mortality Weekly Report* 45.34 (5 June 1981): 729–33; reprint, 30 August 1996.

"Changes in Thai Behavior Lower HIV Spread." *AIDS Weekly Plus*, 2 June 1997, 24ff.

Chartier, Roger. "The Practical Impact of Writing." In *Passions of the Renaissance*, ed. Roger Chartier. Vol. 3 of *A History of Private Life*. Cambridge: Harvard/Belknap, 1989.

Ciavolella, Massimo. *La "malattia d'amore" dall'antichità al medioevo*. Rome: Bulzoni, 1976.

Cipolla, Carlo M. *Public Health and the Medical Profession in the Renaissance*. Cambridge: Cambridge University Press, 1976.

Coates, Thomas J., and Pamela DeCarlo. *We Know What Works in HIV Prevention—Why Aren't We Doing More of It?* San Francisco: Center for AIDS Prevention Studies, UCSF/Harvard AIDS Institute, 1996. Fact sheet.

Cohen, B. D. "Religious Double Standard." *New York Newsday*, 23 February 1993.

Community School Board 24, New York. *Addendum to Notice of Public Meeting—April 28, 1994*. Announcement. Glendale, N.Y.: Community School Board 24, 1994.

Ruelle, Pierre, ed. *Congés d'Arras*. Brussels, 1965.

Congressional Record, 14 October 1987, S 14202–7.

Congressional Record, 20 October 1987, H 8801.

Conyers. "The Politics of AIDS Prevention: Science Takes a Time Out." *Union Calendar*, 102nd Cong., 2nd sess., no. 584, Report 102–1047 (1992): 1–22.

Correll, Alan. "Scientists Linked to the Vatican Call for Population Crisis." *New York Times*, 16 June 1994.

Coulson, Noel J. "Regulation of Sexual Behavior under Traditional Islamic Law." In *Society and the Sexes in Medieval Islam*, ed. Afaf Lufti al-Sayyid-Marsot, 63–68. Malibu, Calif.: Undena, 1979.

Coyecque, Ernest Louis. *L'Hôtel-Dieu de Paris au moyen âge: Histoire et documents*. Paris: H. Champion, 1889–1891.

Crimp, Douglas. *AIDS: Cultural Analysis, Cultural Activism*. Cambridge: MIT Press, 1988.

D., I. *Salomon's Pest-House or Towre-Royall, Newly Re-Edified and Prepared to Preserve Londoners with Their Families, and Others from the Doubted Deluge of the Plague*. 2nd ed. London: For Thomas Harper and Henry Holland, 1630.

Davis, Natalie Zemon. *Society and Culture in Early Modern France: Eight Essays*. Stanford: Stanford University Press, 1975.

DeCarlo, Pamela. *Do Condoms Work?* San Francisco: Center for AIDS Prevention Studies, UCSF/Harvard AIDS Institute, 1995. Fact sheet.

DeCarlo, Pamela, and Thomas Coates. *Does HIV Prevention Work?* San Francisco: Center for AIDS Prevention Studies, 1995. Fact sheet no. 1ER, <http://www.caps.ucsf.edu/preventionrev.html>

Deslandes, Léopold. *Manhood: The Causes of Its Premature Decline, with Directions for Its Perfect Restoration*. 5th ed. Translated by an American Physician. Boston: Otis, Broaders, 1842.

Dickens, Charles. *David Copperfield*. Edited by Nina Burgis. Oxford: Clarendon Press, 1981.

Dickinson, Robert Latou, M.D. "Bicycling for Women from the Standpoint of the Gynecologist." *American Journal of Obstetrics* 31 (1895): 24–37.

Dictionnaire des sciences médicales: Biographie médicale. Paris: C. L. F. Panckoucke, 1820.

Diderot, Denis, and Jean Le Rond d'Alembert, eds. *Encyclopédie, ou, dictionnaire raisonné des sciences, des arts, et des métiers.* 2nd ed. Lucca: Vincent Giuntini, 1758–1771.

———. *Encyclopédie, ou dictionnaire raisonné des sciences, des arts, et des métiers.* 3rd ed. Geneva: J. L. Pettet, 1778–1779.

Dillon, Sam. "Board Removes Fernandez as New York Schools Chief after Stormy 3-Year Term." *New York Times,* 11 February 1993.

Dols, Michael. *The Black Death in the Middle East.* Princeton: Princeton University Press, 1977.

———."Diseases of the Islamic World." In *The Cambridge World History of Human Disease,* ed. Kenneth F. Kiple, 336–8, 338–9. Cambridge: Cambridge University Press, 1993.

———. "The Origins of the Islamic Hospital: Myth and Reality." *Bulletin of the History of Medicine* 61 (1987): 367–90.

Donne, John. *Poems.* Oxford: Oxford University Press, 1912.

Dover, Kenneth James. *Greek Homosexuality.* Cambridge: Harvard University Press, 1978.

Dreisbach, Robert H., and William O. Robertson. *Handbook of Poisoning.* 12th ed. Norwalk, Conn.: Appleton and Lange, 1987.

Du Breul, Jacques. *Le theatre des antiquitez de Paris, ou est traicté de la fondation des églises & chapelles de la cité, université, ville, & diocese de Paris.* Paris: Société des Imprimeurs, 1639.

Duane, Thomas K. [Council member, 3rd District, Manhattan]. Letter to Richard Yezzo, President, St. Clare's Hospital. New York City Council, 22 February 1994.

Dubé, M. *Le médecin et le chirurgien des pauvres.* 5th ed. Paris: Couterot, 1678.

Edelheit, Joseph A. Lecture, "AIDS: A Transformative Challenge for Clergy." N.p., n.d.

Editorial, "Civil Disobedience vs. Uncivilized Behavior." *New York Daily News,* 12 December 1989.

Editorial, "'Family Values' Won't Save Our Youth." *Our Town* (New York), 27 January 1994.

Editorial, "Little Ad-Vantage to This Campaign." *New York Daily News,* 30 January 1994.

Editorial, "More Gay-Bashing." *Nation,* 31 October 1987.

Editorial, "Porn Rides the Rails." *New York Post,* 20 January 1994.

Editorial, "Sacrilege in St. Pat's." *New York Post,* 12 December 1989.

Editorial, "Some Hope on Third-World AIDS." *New York Times,* 7 October 1996.

Editorial, "The Storming of St. Pat's." *New York Times,* 12 December 1989.

Editorial, "What the Doctor Ordered." *Moody Monthly,* October 1988, 12.

Editorial, "What Mr. Bush Can Do on AIDS." *New York Times,* 10 December 1991.

Elders, Joycelyn, and David Chanoff. *Joycelyn Elders, M.D.: From Sharecropper's Daughter to Surgeon General of the United States of America.* New York: William Morrow and Co., 1996.

Ell, Stephen R. "Blood and Sexuality in Medieval Leprosy." *Janus* 7 (1984): 153–64.

Elliott, Dyan. "Pollution, Illusion, and Masculine Disarray: Nocturnal Emissions and the Sexuality of the Clergy." In *Constructing Medieval Sexuality,* ed. Peggy McCracken, Karma Lochrie, and James A. Schultz. Minneapolis: University of Minnesota Press, 1997.

Ellis, Havelock. "Autoerotism." In *Studies in the Psychology of Sex,* 3: 110–204. 7 vols. Philadelphia: F. A. Davis, 1900–1917.

Elton, G. R. *Reformation Europe.* New York: Harper and Row, 1963.

Emmison, F. G. *Elizabethan Life: Morals and the Church Courts.* Chelmsford: Essex County Council, 1973.

Engelhardt, Tristram. "The Disease of Masturbation: Values and Concepts of Disease." *Bulletin of the History of Medicine* 48 (1974): 234–48.

Epstein, Julia. *Altered Conditions: Disease, Medicine, and Storytelling.* New York: Routledge, 1994.

Erasmus, Desiderius. "Inns." In *Colloquies of Erasmus,* ed. Craig Thompson. Chicago: University of Chicago Press, 1965.

———. "A Marriage in Name Only." In *Colloquies of Erasmus,* ed. Craig Thompson. Chicago: University of Chicago Press, 1965.

Estes, J. Worth. *Dictionary of Protopharmacology: Therapeutic Practices, 1700–1850.* Canton, Mass.: Science History Publications, 1990.

Fallopius, Girolamo. *De morbo gallico liber absolutissimus.* Padua: Luca Bertellus, 1564.

Falwell, Jerry. "AIDS, the Judgment of God." *Liberty Report* (Lynchburg, Va.: Moral Majority Foundation), April 1987, 2, 5.

Farah, Madelain, ed. and trans. *Marriage and Sexuality in Islam: A Translation of Al-Ghazāli's Book on the Etiquette of Marriage from the Ihyā'.* Salt Lake City: University of Utah Press, 1984.

Fay, Henri Marcel. *Histoire de la lèpre en France: Lépreux et cagots du Sud-Ouest: Notes historiques, médicales, philologiques, suivies de documents par le Dr. H. M. Fay, avec une préface du Professeur Gilbert Ballet.* Paris: Librairie ancienne Honoré Champion, 1910.

Feder, Don. "How Tax Dollars Help Pay for Instruction in the Homosexual Way of Sex." *New York Post,* 9 November 1987.

———. "YUK! 92 U.S. Senators Feel the Same Way." *Minneapolis Daily American,* 25 November 1987.

Federal Security Agency, Social Security Administration. *Infant Care.* Children's Bureau Publication no. 8. Washington, D.C.: Goverment Printing Office, 1951.

Fernandez, Joseph, with John Underwood. *Tales out of School: Joseph Fernandez's Crusade to Rescue American Education.* Boston: Little, Brown, 1993.

Ferrand, Jacques. *A Treatise on Lovesickness.* Edited and translated by Donald A. Beecher and Massimo Ciavolella. Syracuse, N.Y.: Syracuse University Press, 1990.

Fineberg, Harvey V. "Education to Prevent AIDS: Prospects and Obstacles." *Science* 239 (5 February 1988): 592–6.

Fletcher, James. "Homosexuality: Kick and Kickback." *Southern Medical Journal* 77.2 (February 1984): 149–50.

"Follow the Facts: Condoms Work, Distortions Don't." *New York Newsday,* 18 May 1994.

Foucault, Michel. *The History of Sexuality.* Translated by Robert Hurley. 3 vols. New York: Vintage Books, 1985.

Fouquet, Marie de Maupeou, *Recueil de remedes faciles et domestiques, choisis, experimentez & tres-approuvés, pour toute sorte de maladies, internes & externes, inveterées & difficiles à guerir. Recueillis par les ordres charitables d'une illustre & pieuse Dame, pour soulager les pauvres malades.* Dijon: Ressayre, 1678.

Fout, John. *Forbidden History: The State, Society, and the Regulation of Sexuality in Early Modern Europe.* Chicago: University of Chicago Press, 1992.

Fracastorius, Hieronymus. "De syphilide, seu morbo gallico lucubratio." In *De morbo gallico omnia quae extant apud omnes medicos cuiuscunque nationis,* ed. Aloysius Luisinus. Venice: S. Zilettus, 1563.

Fracastoro, Girolamo. *De contagione et contagiosis morbis et eorum curatione libri III.* Translated by Wilmer C. Wright. New York: Putnam's Sons, 1930.

Freud, Sigmund. "Contributions to a Discussion on Masturbation." In *Standard Edition of the Complete Psychological Works of Sigmund Freud,* ed. James Strachey, 12: 239–54. London: Hogarth Press, 1938 [1912].

———. *Three Contributions to the Theory of Sex.* 3rd ed. Translated by A. A. Brill. New York: Nervous and Mental Disease Publishing Co., 1918 [1905].

Friedman, Saul. "Presidential Advice on AIDS Prevention." *New York Newsday,* 2 April 1987.

Fuchs, Josef. *Natural Law: A Theological Investigation.* Translated by Helmut Reckter and John A. Dowling. New York: Sheed and Ward, 1965.

Fumento, Michael. *The Myth of Heterosexual AIDS. How a Tragedy Has Been Distorted by the Media and Partisan Politics.* Washington D.C.: Regency Gateway, 1993.

Galen, Claudius. "De locis affectis." In *Claudii Galeni opera omnia.* Vol. 8 of *Medicorum graecorum opera quae extant,* ed. C. G. Kuhn. Hildesheim: Georg Olms, 1965.

———. *Galen on the Affected Parts.* Translated by Rudolph E. Siegel. Munich: S. Karger, 1976.

Garrett, Laurie. *The Coming Plague: Newly Emerging Diseases in a World out of Balance.* New York: Farrar, Straus and Giroux, 1994.

"Gay Comic." *Washington Times,* 8 October 1987.

Gay Men's Health Crisis et al. v. Dr. Louis Sullivan and James O. Mason. United States District

Court, Southern District of New York. 88 Civ. 7482 (SWK). *Plaintiffs' Memorandum of Law in Support of Partial Summary Judgment and in Opposition to Defendants' Motion to Dismiss or for Summary Judgment.*

Geremek, Bronisław. *The Margins of Society in Late Medieval Paris.* Translated by Jean Birrell. Cambridge: Cambridge University Press, 1987.

Gerson, Jean. *De cognitione castitatis et pollutionibus diurnis, cum forma absolutionis.* Cologne: Ulrich Zel, 1470–1472.

———. *De confessione molliciei.* Vol. 2 of *Opera,* sec. 33. Basel: Nicolaus Kesler, 1489.

Gilbert, Arthur N. "Doctor, Patient, and Onanist Diseases in the Nineteenth Century." *Journal of the History of Medicine and Allied Sciences* 30 (1975): 217–34.

Gilinus, Conradinus. "De morbo quem gallicum nuncupant." In *The Earliest Printed Literature on Syphilis,* ed. Karl Sudhoff. Florence: R. Lier, 1925.

Gillispie, Charles Coulston, ed. *Dictionary of Scientific Biography.* New York: Charles Scribner's Sons, 1980.

GMHC v. Sullivan. See *Gay Men's Health Crisis.*

Goitein, S. D. "The Sexual Mores of the Common People." In *Society and the Sexes in Medieval Islam,* ed. Afaf Lufti al-Sayyid-Marsot, 43–61. Malibu, Calif.: Undena, 1979.

Goldman, Ari L. "Episcopal Bishop Criticizes Catholic Church." *New York Times,* 1 April 1992.

———. "U.S. Bishops Back Condom Education as a Move on AIDS." *New York Times,* 11 December 1987.

Gollmann, Wilhelm. *The Homeopathic Guide: In All Diseases of the Urinary and Sexual Organs, Including the Derangements Caused by Onanism and Sexual Excesses. . . .* Translated by M.D. Chas. J. Hempel. Philadelphia: Rademacher and Sheek, 1855.

Goodman, Lawrence. "Catholic Group to Explode Condom Secret." *New York Post,* 27 April 1994.

Gordon, Bernard de. *Lilium medicinae.* Lyons: G. Rouillium, 1550.

Grimm, Harold J. "Luther's Contribution to Sixteenth-Century Organization of Poor Relief." *Archive for Reformation History* 61–2 (1970): 222–33.

Grünpeck, J. *Tractatus de pestilentiali scorra und hübscher Tractat von dem Ursprung des Bösen Franzos.* In *The Earliest Printed Literature on Syphilis,* ed. Karl Sudhoff. Florence: R. Lier, 1925.

Guardian Family Association. Advertisement. *New York Post,* 22 March 1993.

Gutton, Jean-Pierre. "L'enfermement à l'âge classique." In *Histoire des hôpitaux en France,* ed. Jean Imbert, 161–94. Toulouse: Privat, 1982.

———. "Hôtels-Dieu et hôpitaux de malades à l'âge classique (XVIIe–XVIIIe siècles)." In *Histoire des hôpitaux en France,* ed. Jean Imbert, 195–220. Toulouse: Privat, 1982.

———. "Mutations." In *Histoire des hôpitaux en France,* ed. Jean Imbert. Toulouse: Privat, 1982.

Hall, G. Stanley. *Adolescence: Its Psychology and Its Relations to Physiology, Anthropology, Sociology, Sex, Crime, Religion, and Education.* 2 vols. New York: D. Appleton and Co., 1904.

Hall, Lesley L. "Forbidden by God, Despised by Men: Masturbation, Medical Warnings, Moral Panic, and Manhood in Great Britain, 1850–1950." In *Forbidden History,* ed. John Fout, 293–315. Chicago: University of Chicago Press, 1992.

Hall, Winfried Scott, M.D. *Sexual Knowledge: The Knowledge of Self and Sex in Simple Language.* Philadelphia: John C. Winston, 1916.

———. *The Strength of Ten: What Manhood Is, and How a Boy May Win It.* La Crosse, Wisc.: B. Steadwell, 1912.

Halperin, David M. *One Hundred Years of Homosexuality and Other Essays on Greek Love.* New York: Routledge, 1989.

Halperin, David M., John J. Winkler, and Froma Zeitlin, eds. *Before Sexuality: The Construction of Erotic Experience in the Ancient Greek World.* Princeton: Princeton University Press, 1990.

Harden, Victoria A., and Guenter B. Risse. *AIDS and the Historian.* Proceedings of a Conference at the National Institutes of Health, 20–21 March 1989. NIH Publication no. 91–1584. [Bethesda, Md.]: U.S. Department of Health and Human Services, Public Health Service, National Institutes of Health, 1991.

Hare, E. H. "Masturbational Insanity: The History of an Idea." *Journal of Mental Science* 108 (1962): 2–25.

Harvey, E. Ruth. *The Inward Wits: Psychological Theory in the Middle Ages and the Renaissance.* London: Warburg Institute, University of London, 1975.

Harvey, Gideon. *The Family Physician, and the House Apothecary.* London: T. R[ookes?], 1671.

————. *Great Venus Unmasked: Or a More Exact Discovery of the Venereal Evil, or French Disease, Comprizing the Opinions of Most Ancient and Modern Physicians, with the Particular Sentiment of the Author Touching the Rise, Nature, Subject, Causes, Kinds, Progress, Changes, Signs, and Prognosticks of the Said Evil, Together with Luculent Problems, Pregnant Observations, and the Most Practical Cures of That Disease, and Virulent Gonorrhoea, or Running of the Reins. Likewise a Tract of General Principles of Physick, with Discourses of the Scurvy, Manginess, and Plague.* London: B. G. for Nath. Brook, 1672.

Heitzberg, Arthur. "Catholics, Jews, and the Abortion Debate." *Reform Judaism* (Winter 1996).

Herring, Francis. *Preservatives against the Plague or Directions and Advertisements for This Time of Pestilential Contagion, with Certain Instructions for the Poorer Sort of People When They Shall Be Visited; and Also a Caveat to Those That Were [sic] about Their Necks Imprisoned Amulets as a Preservative against That Sickness.* London: for Thomas Pierrepont, 1665.

Hexter, Ralph J. *Ovid and Medieval Schooling: Studies in Medieval School Commentaries on Ovid's* Ars amatoria, Epistulae ex Ponto, *and* Epistulae heroidum. Munich: Arbeo-Gesellschaft, 1986.

Hildegard von Bingen. *Causae et curae.* Edited by P. Kaiser. Biblioteca scriptorum graecorum et romanorum teubneriana, 133. Leipzig: Teubner, 1903.

Holmes, King K., ed. *Sexually Transmitted Diseases.* 2nd ed. New York: McGraw-Hill, 1990.

Hoveden, Roger de. *The Annals of Roger de Hoveden, Containing the History of England and of Other Countries of Europe from* A.D. *732 to* A.D. *1201.* Translated by Henry T. Riley. 2 vols. London: H. G. Bohn, 1853; reprint, New York: AMS Press, 1968.

Hutchinson, Jonathan. "On Circumcision as Preventive of Masturbation." *Archives of Surgery* 2 (1891): 267.

Hutten, Ulrich von. *Of the Wood Called Guiacum, That Healeth the French Pockes, and Also Helpeth the Goute in the Feete, the Stone, Palsey, Lepre, Dropsy, Fallynge Evyl, and Other Diseases.* Translated by Thomas Paynel. London: Thomas Berthelet, 1540.

Imbert, Jean. *Les hôpitaux en droit canonique.* Paris, 1947.

————. *Les hôpitaux en France.* Paris: Presses Universitaires de France, 1958.

Jacquart, Danielle, and Françoise Micheau. *La médecine arabe et l'Occident médiéval.* Paris: Maisonneuve et Larose, 1990.

Jacquart, Danielle, and Claude Thomasset. *Sexuality and Medicine in the Middle Ages.* Translated by Matthew Adamson. Princeton: Princeton University Press, 1988.

Jacque, Dr. "Société de chirurgerie: Séance du mercredi 13 janvier 1864." *L'union médicale,* n.s. 21 (1864): 91–5.

James, Edward T., et al. *Dictionary of American Biography,* suppl. 3 *(1941–1945).* New York: Charles Scribner's Sons, 1973.

Janison, Dan. "Pols All Hot and Bothered by Subway AIDS Ads." *New York Post,* 28 January 1994.

Jean de Saint-Amand (Johannes de Sancto Amando). *Concordanciae.* Edited by Julius Leopold Pagel. Berlin: G. Reimer, 1894.

Jeanselme, Edouard. *Comment l'Europe, au moyen âge, se protégea contre la lèpre.* Brussels: Imprimerie médicale et scientifique, 1930.

Johnson, Allen, ed. *Dictionary of American Biography.* 20 vols. New York: Charles Scribner's Sons, 1928.

Johnston, William D. "Tuberculosis." In *The Cambridge World History of Human Diseases,* ed. Kenneth F. Kiple, 1059–67. Cambridge: Cambridge University Press, 1993.

Jones, Ernest, M.D. *Papers on Psycho-Analysis.* 2nd ed. New York: William Wood, 1919 [1912].

Jones, Richard Foster. *Ancients and Moderns: A Study of the Rise of the Scientific Movement in Seventeenth-Century England.* St. Louis, Mo.: Washington University, 1961.

Jonsen, Albert R., and Jeff Stryker. *The Social Impact of AIDS in the United States.* Washington D.C.: National Academy Press, 1993.

Jordanova, Ludmilla. "The Popularisation of Medicine: Tissot on Onanism." *Textual Practice* 1 (1987): 68–80.

Joubert, Laurent. *Erreurs populaires et propos vulgaires, touchant la médecine et le régime de santé.* Bourdeaux: S. Millanges, 1579.

Kahn, James G., and Pamela DeCarlo. *Is HIV Prevention a Good Investment?* San Francisco: Center for AIDS Prevention Studies, UCSF/Harvard AIDS Institute, 1995. Fact sheet.

Kaplan, Harold I., and Benjamin J. Sadock. *Comprehensive Textbook of Psychiatry/VI.* 6th ed. 2 vols. Baltimore: Williams and Wilkins, 1995.

Kellogg, John Harvey, M.D. *Plain Facts for Young and Old.* Reprint, New York: Arno Press, 1974 [1886].

Kelly, Howard A., and Walter L. Burrage. *Dictionary of American Medical Biography.* Boston: Milford House, 1971.

Kerrison, Ray. "Sleazy AIDS Ads Take the Gay Train." *New York Post,* 19 January 1994.

Kilpatrick, James. "It's Encouraging Safe Sodomy." *San Antonio (Texas) Express and News,* 18 November 1987.

———. "Should Our Taxes Promote Safe Sodomy?" *Seattle Daily Times,* 19 December 1987.

Kingdon, Robert M. "Social Welfare in Calvin's Geneva." *American Historical Review* 76.1 (1971): 50–69.

Kinsey, Alfred C., and Wardell B. Pomeroy. *Sexual Behavior in the Human Male.* Philadelphia: W. B. Saunders and Co., 1948.

Kinsey, Alfred C., et al. *Sexual Behavior in the Human Female.* Philadelphia: W. B. Saunders Company, 1953.

Kiple, Kenneth F. *The Cambridge World History of Human Disease.* Cambridge: Cambridge University Press, 1993.

Kirkbride, Thomas, M.D. *Reports of the Pennsylvania Hospital for the Insane, 1841–1850.* Philadelphia: Pennsylvania Hospital, 1851.

Koenigsberger, H. G., and, George L. Mosse. *Europe in the Sixteenth Century.* London: Longmans, Green and Co., 1968.

Kolata, Gina. "Congress, NIH, Open for AIDS." *Science,* 29 July 1983, 436.

Koop, C. Everett. *Koop: The Memoirs of America's Family Doctor.* New York: Random House, 1991.

Krafft-Ebing, Richard von. *Psychopathia sexualis.* Philadelphia: F. A. Davis, 1892.

Lambert, Bruce. "A Church-State Conflict Arises over AIDS Care." *New York Times,* March 1990.

Lawrence, Edward. *Christ's Power over Bodily Diseases Preached in Several Sermons on Mat. 8. 5, 6, 7, 8, 9, 10, 11, 12, 13, and Published for the Instruction, Especially of the More Ignorant People, in the Great Duty of Preparation for Sickness and Death.* London: R. W. for Francis Tyton, 1662.

Lebrun, François. *Se soigner autrefois: Médecins, saints, et sorciers aux 17e et 18e siècles.* Paris: Les Temps Actuels, 1983.

Lee, Sidney, ed. *Dictionary of National Biography.* New York: Macmillan and Co., 1892.

LeGrand, Léon. *Statuts d'Hôtels-Dieu et de léproseries; Recueil de textes du XIIe au XIVe siècle.* Collection de textes pour servir à l'étude et à l'enseignement de l'histoire 29. Paris: A. Picard, 1901.

Leonard, E. M. *The Early History of English Poor Relief.* London: Frank Cass and Co., 1965.

Léonard, Jacques. *La France médicale: Médecins et malades au XIXe siècle.* Paris: Gallimard, 1978.

Liébault, Jean. *Thrésor des remedes secrets pour les maladies des femmes.* Paris: Jacques du Puys, 1587.

London's Lamentation, Or a Fit Admonishment for City and Countrey, Wherein Is Described Certain Causes of This Affliction and Visitation of the Plague, Yeare 1641, Which the Lord Hath Been Pleased to Inflict upon Us, and Withall What Meanes Must Be Used to the Lord, to Gaine His Mercy and Favor, with an Excellent Spirituall Medicine to Be Used for the Preservation Both of Body and Soule. London: E. P. for John Wright Junior, 1641.

Long, Harland William, M.D. *Sane Sex Life and Sane Sex Living: Some Things That All Sane People Ought to Know.* Boston: Richard G. Badger, 1919.

Luther, Martin. "A Sermon on the Estate of Marriage." In *Basic Theological Writings of Martin Luther*, ed. Timothy F. Lull, 630–7. Minneapolis: Fortress Press, 1989.

―――. "Whether One May Flee from a Deadly Plague." In *Basic Theological Writings of Martin Luther*, ed. Timothy F. Lull, 736–55. Minneapolis, Minn.: Fortress Press, 1989.

MacDonald, Robert H. "The Frightful Consequences of Onanism: Notes on the History of a Delusion." *Journal of the History of Ideas* 27 (1967): 423–31.

Mangaliman, Jessie. "Ads on Two Tracks: Dueling Posters Put Views on Condoms into the Subways." *New York Newsday*, 18 May 1994.

Mann, Jonathan, Daniel J. M. Tarantola, and Thomas W. Netter, eds. *AIDS in the World: A Global Report*. Cambridge: Harvard University Press, 1992.

Mann, Ronald D. *Modern Drug Use: An Enquiry on Historical Principles*. Boston: MTP Press, 1984.

Marquis Who's Who. http://web-lexis-nexis.com/universe/doc: Reed Elsevier Inc., accessed 3 May 1998.

Martin, William C. *With God on Our Side: The Rise of the Religious Right in America*. New York: Broadway Books, 1996.

Marty, Martin, and R. Scott Appleby. *The Glory and the Power: The Fundamentalist Challenge to the Modern World*. Boston: Beacon Press, 1992.

Massa, Nicolas. "De morbo gallico liber." In *De morbo gallico omnia quae extant apud omnes medicos cuiuscunque nationis*, ed. Aloysius Luisinus. Venice: S. Zilettus, 1563.

Mather, Cotton. *The Angel of Bethesda*. Edited by Gordon W. Jones. Worcester, Mass.: American Antiquarian Society and Barre Publishers, 1974 [1724].

Matlick, Maralyn. "Backlash-Wary Gays Rip Protest at St. Pat's." *New York Post*, 13 December 1989.

Maubray, John. *The Female Physician, Containing All the Diseases Incident to That Sex, in Virgins, Wives, and Widows. . . .* London: Stephen Austen, 1730.

Mayes, J. A. "Spermatorrhoea Treated by the Lately Invented Rings." *Charleston Medical Journal and Review* 9 (1854): 351–3.

McDowell, Josh. "The Teen Sex Crisis." *Religious Broadcasting*, January 1987, 16–18.

McIlhaney, Joe S. Fundraising letter for the Medical Institute for Sexual Health.

McKernan, Kathleen. "Huntington Man Gets 4 Years; Defendant Tells Court He Performed Surgeries in Order to Help People." *Indianapolis Star*, April 13, 1999.

McNeill, John T., and Helena M. Gamer. *Medieval Handbooks of Penance*. New York: Columbia University Press, 1938.

Medical Institute for Sexual Health. *The Facts about the STD Epidemic*. Austin, Tex.: Medical Institute for Sexual Health, 1996. Pamphlet.

Mercier, Charles Arthur. *Leper Houses and Medieval Hospitals*. Fitzpatrick lectures, 1914. London: H. K. Lewis, 1915.

Metropolitan Community Church. *AIDS: Is It God's Judgment?* Los Angeles: Metropolitan Community Church, n.d. Pamphlet.

Miller, Timothy S. *The Birth of the Hospital in the Byzantine Empire*. Baltimore: Johns Hopkins University Press, 1985.

Milton, John Laws. *On Spermatorrhea: Its Pathology, Results, and Complications*. 11th ed. London: Renshaw, 1881.

Modras, Ronald. "Pope John Paul II's Theology of the Body." In *The Vatican and Homosexuality*, ed. Jeannine Gramick and Pat Furey, 119–25. New York: Crossroad, 1988.

Mollat, Michel. "Dans la perspective de l'au-delà (XIVe–XVe siècles)." In *Histoire des hôpitaux en France*, ed. Jean Imbert, 67–96. Toulouse: Privat, 1982.

―――. "Floraison des fondations hospitalières, XIIe–XIIIe siècles." In *Histoire des hôpitaux en France*, ed. Jean Imbert, 33–66. Toulouse: Privat, 1982.

―――. "La vie quotidienne dans les hôpitaux médiévaux." In *Histoire des hôpitaux en France*, ed. Jean Imbert, 97–134. Toulouse: Privat, 1982.

————. "Les premiers hôpitaux (VIe–XIe siècles)." In *Histoire des hôpitaux en France*, ed. Jean Imbert, 13–32. Toulouse: Privat, 1982.

Montesauro, N. *De dispositionibus, quas vulgares mal franzoso appellant.* In *The Earliest Printed Works on Syphilis*, ed. Karl Sudhoff. Florence: Florence: R. Lier, 1925.

Mooney, Mark. "Commish Slams Anti-Condom Ads." *New York Daily News*, 23 May 1994.

Murphy, Timothy F. *Ethics in an Epidemic: AIDS, Morality, and Culture.* Berkeley: University of California Press, 1994.

Myers, Steven Lee. "Queens School Board Suspended in Fight on Gay-Life Curriculum." *New York Times*, 2 December 1992.

"The Nation's Most Common Infections Are Sexual."*New York Times*, 20 October 1996.

Navarro, Mireya. "Group Begins New AIDS Ads in Subways." *New York Times*, 14 January 1994.

Nicholson, Joe. "AIDS Epidemic Just Got Wor$e." *New York Post*, 30 December 1992.

————. "Bishop Pulls Plug on State AIDS Book." *New York Post*, 19 September 1992.

Niebuhr, Gustav. "Week in Review: Kneeling at the Altar of Death: From Belief to Fanaticism." *New York Times*, 14 August 1994, 5.

Nikiforuk, Andrew. *The Fourth Horseman: A Short History of Epidemics, Plagues, Famine and Other Scourges.* New York: M. Evans and Co., 1993.

Nirenberg, David. *Communities of Violence: Persecution of Minorities in the Middle Ages.* Princeton: Princeton University Press, 1996.

Nutton, Vivian. "From Galen to Alexander: Aspects of Medicine and Medical Practice in Late Antiquity." In *Symposium on Byzantine Medicine*, ed. John Scarborough, 1–14. Dumbarton Oaks Papers, 38. Washington, D.C.: Dumbarton Oaks, 1983.

"O'Connor: Spiritual Focus Needed." *Newsday* [1987].

Office of Technology Assessment. *How Effective Is AIDS Education?* Staff paper no. 3. Washington D.C.: Office of Technology Assessment, 1988.

Onania, or the Heinous Sin of Self-Pollution, and All Its Frightful Consequences, in Both Sexes, Considered. 10th ed. Boston: John Phillips, 1724.

O'Neill, Ynez Violé. "Diseases of the Middle Ages." In *The Cambridge World History of Human Disease*, ed. Kenneth F. Kiple, 270–9. Cambridge: Cambridge University Press, 1993.

Pagel, Walter. *Paracelsus: An Introduction to Philosophical Medicine in the Era of the Renaissance.* New York: Karger, 1982.

Papers of Conference on "Sexual Abstinence and Its Effects on Health." *Zeitschrift für Bekämpfung der Geschlechtskrankheiten* 13 (1911).

Paré, Ambroise. *The Workes of That Famous Chirurgion Ambrose Parey.* Translated by Tho. Johnson. London: Richard Cotes and William Du-gard, 1649.

Park, Katharine. "Black Death." In *The Cambridge World History of Human Disease*, ed. Kenneth F. Kiple, 612–6. Cambridge: Cambridge University Press, 1993.

————. *Doctors and Medicine in Early Renaissance Florence.* Princeton: Princeton University Press, 1985.

————. "Healing the Poor: Hospitals and Medical Assistance in Renaissance Florence." In *Medicine and Charity before the Welfare State*, ed. Jonathan Barry and Colin Jones, 26–45. London: Routledge, 1991.

————. "Medicine and Society in Medieval Europe, 500–1500." In *Medicine in Society: Historical Essays*, ed. Andrew Wear, 59–90. New York: Cambridge University Press, 1992.

Parsons, Gail Pat. "Equal Treatment for All: American Medical Remedies for Male Sexual Problems 1850–1900." *Journal of the History of Medicine and Allied Sciences* 32.1 (1977): 55–71.

Partner, Nancy. "Making Up Lost Time: Writing on the Writing of History." *Speculum* 61.1 (January 1986).

Payer, Pierre J. *The Bridling of Desire: Views of Sex in the Later Middle Ages.* Toronto: University of Toronto Press, 1993.

Pennington, D. H. *Europe in the Seventeenth Century.* 2nd ed. London: Longman, 1989.

Pennsylvania Hospital. *150th Annual Report of the Board of Managers: Department for the Sick and*

190   BIBLIOGRAPHY

Wounded, and Departments for the Insane, May 1900–May 1901. Philadelphia: T. C. Davis and Sons, 1901.
Pennsylvania Hospital Case Books, Old Style. Philadelphia: Pennsylvania Hospital, 1841.
Pennsylvania Hospital Reports. Philadelphia: Pennsylvania Hospital, 1873–1874.
Perrot, Michelle, ed. *From the Fires of Revolution to the Great War.* Translated by Arthur Goldhammer. Vol. 4 of *A History of Private Life,* ed. Philippe Ariès and Georges Duby. Cambridge: Harvard/Belknap, 1990.
Perrow, Charles, and Mauro F. Guillen. *The AIDS Disaster: The Failure of Organizations in New York and the Nation.* New Haven: Yale University Press, 1990.
Peter of Spain (Petrus Hispanus, later Pope John XXI). *Thesaurus pauperum* (Treasure chest of the poor). In *Practica Jo. Serapionis,* ff. 253–72. Lyons: Jacob Myt, 1525.
Petit, Marc-Antoine. *Onan, ou, le tombeau du Mont-cindre . . . présenté en 1809 à l'Académie des jeux floraux de Toulouse.* Lyons: J. B. Kindelem, 1809.
Plarr, Victor Gustave. *Plarr's Lives of the Fellows of the Royal College of Surgeons of England.* London: Royal College of Surgeons, 1930.
Porter, Dorothy, and Roy Porter. *Patient's Progress: The Dialectics of Doctoring in Eighteenth-Century England.* Cambridge: Cambridge University Press, 1989.
Porter, Roy. *English Society in the Eighteenth Century.* London: Penguin, 1990.
———. "Forbidden Pleasures: Enlightenment Literature of Sexual Advice." In *Solitary Pleasures,* ed. Paula Bennett and Vernon A. Rosario, 75–98. New York: Routledge, 1995.
———. Introduction to *Sexual Knowledge, Sexual Science: The History of Attitudes to Sexuality,* ed. Roy Porter and Mikulas Teich, 1–26. Cambridge: Cambridge University Press, 1994.
"Prevention May Cut AIDS Toll." *New York Daily News,* 8 August 1995.
Pseudo-Aristotle. *Aristotle's Master-Piece.* London: D. P., 1720.
Quétel, Claude. *History of Syphilis.* Translated by Judith Braddock and Brian Pike. Baltimore: Johns Hopkins University Press, 1990.
Quindlen, Anna. "Public and Private: Church and State." *New York Times,* 17 February 1993.
Ratzinger, Cardinal Joseph. Congregation for the Doctrine of Faith."Letter to the Bishops of the Catholic Church on the Pastoral Care of Homosexual Persons." In *The Vatican and Homosexuality,* ed. Jeannine Gramick and Pat Furey, 1–10. New York: Crossroad, 1988.
"Ray of Hope in Uganda in War against HIV." *AIDS Weekly Plus,* 3 March 1997, 19ff.
Reuter. "Buchanan: AIDS Is 'Retribution.'" *New York Newsday,* 28 February 1992.
Rhazes. *Al-Hawi Fi'l-Tibb (Liber continentis in medicina).* Brescia: Jacobus Britannicus, 1486.
Richards, Peter. *The Medieval Leper and His Northern Heirs.* Cambridge and Totowa, N.J.: D. S. Brewer and Rowman and Littlefield, 1977.
Richardson, Jeff. Letter to the editor. *New York Daily News,* 14 February 1994.
———. Letter to the editor. *New York Post,* 29 January 1994.
Risse, Guenter B. "History of Western Medicine from Hippocrates to Germ Theory." In *The Cambridge World History of Human Disease,* ed. Kenneth F. Kiple, 11–9. Cambridge: Cambridge University Press, 1993.
Roan, Shari. "When the Church and Medicine Clash." *Los Angeles Times,* 2 February 1995.
Rosario, Vernon A. "Phantastical Pollutions: The Public Threat of Private Vice in France." In *Solitary Pleasures,* ed. Paula Bennett and Vernon A. Rosario, 101–30. New York: Routledge, 1995.
Rossiaud, Jacques. *Medieval Prostitution.* Translated by Lydia G. Cochrane. Oxford: Basil Blackwell, 1988.
Rotello, Gabriel. *Sexual Ecology: AIDS and the Destiny of Gay Men.* New York: Dutton, 1997.
Rothenberg, Richard B. "Gonorrhea." In *The Cambridge World History of Human Diseases,* ed. Kenneth F. Kiple, 756–63. Cambridge: Cambridge University Press, 1993.
Rush, Benjamin, M.D. *Medical Inquiries and Observations upon Diseases of the Mind.* Philadelphia: Kimber and Richardson, 1812.
S., L. *ΠΡΟΦΥΛΑΚΤΙΚΟΝ (Prophylaktikon), Or, Some Considerations of a Notable Expedient to*

Root Out the French Pox from the English Nation, with Excellent Defensive Remedies to Preserve Mankind from the Infection of Pocky Women. London [n.p.], 1673.

Sachaile, C. *Les médecins de Paris.* Paris: C. Sachaile, 1845.

Sadler, John. *Enchiridion medicum: An Enchiridion of the Art of Physick.* Translated by R[obert] T[urner]. London: J. C. for R. Moone and Henry Fletcher, 1657.

Schellig, Conradus. *In pustulas malas quem malum de Francia vulgus appellat consilium.* In *The Earliest Printed Literature on Syphilis,* ed. Karl Sudhoff. Florence: R. Lier, 1925.

Schietinger, Helen. *Good Intentions: A Report on Federal HIV Prevention Programs.* Washington, D.C.: AIDS Action Council, 1991.

"School Parents Call Halt to Use of Book on AIDS." *New York Times,* 14 March 1996.

Schwarz, J. C. *Who's Who among Physicians and Surgeons.* New York, 1938.

Shepard, D. "The Cost of AIDS: Prevention and Education." *World Health* 50.5 (1997): 20ff.

Shilts, Randy. *And The Band Played On: Politics, People, and the AIDS Epidemic.* New York: Penguin, 1988.

Sider, Ronald J. "AIDS: An Evangelical Perspective." *Christian Century* 105.1 (6 January 1998).

Simpson, James Young. "Antiquarian Notices of Leprosy and Leper Hospitals in Scotland and England." *Edinburgh Medical and Surgical Journal* [pt. 1] 56 (1841): 301–30; [pt. 2] 57 (1842): 121–56, 394–429.

———. *Antiquarian Notices of Syphilis in Scotland in the Fifteenth and Sixteenth Centuries.* Edinburgh: Edmonston and Douglas, 1862.

Siraisi, Nancy G. *Medieval and Early Renaissance Medicine: An Introduction to Knowledge and Practice.* Chicago: University of Chicago Press, 1990.

Slack, Paul. *The Impact of Plague on Tudor and Stuart England.* London: Routledge and Kegan Paul, 1985.

———. "Mortality Crises and Epidemic Disease in England, 1485–1610." In *Health, Medicine, and Mortality in the Sixteenth Century,* ed. Charles Webster, 9–60. Cambridge: Cambridge University Press, 1979.

Smith, Richard L. *AIDS, Gays, and the American Catholic Church.* Cleveland, Ohio: Pilgrim Press, 1994.

Spitz, René. "Authority and Masturbation: Some Remarks on a Bibliographical Investigation." *Yearbook of Psychoanalysis* 9 (1953): 113–45.

Steinfels, Peter. "Catholic Bishops Vote to Retain Controversial Statement on AIDS." *New York Times,* 28 June 1988.

———. "Southern Baptists Won't Give Out Surgeon General's Report on AIDS." *New York Times,* 23 September 1988.

Steinhardt, Irving David, M.D. *Ten Sex Talks to Boys.* Philadelphia: J. B. Lippincott Co., 1914.

Stekel, Wilhelm. *Auto-Erotism: A Psychiatric Study of Onanism and Neurosis.* Translated by James S. van Teslaar. New York: Liveright, 1950.

———. *Onanie und Homosexualität.* 3rd ed. Berlin: Urban and Schwarzenberg, 1923.

Stengers, Jean, and Anne Van Neck. *Histoire d'une grande peur: La masturbation.* Brussels: Editions de l'Université de Bruxelles, 1984.

Stephen, Leslie, ed. *Dictionary of National Biography.* 63 vols. New York: Macmillan and Co., 1886.

Stevens, Linda. "Cardinal Is Top Speaker on AIDS." *New York Post,* 13 November 1989.

Stevens, Linda, and Rocco Parascandola. "Protests Rock St. Pat's: 111 Arrested in Protest Rally at Cathedral." *New York Post,* 11 December 1989.

Stevens, Linda, and Richard Stein. "O'Connor Digs In." *New York Post,* 12 December 1989.

Stone, Lee Alexander, M.D. *It Is Sex O'Clock.* Chicago: Marshall Field Annex, 1928.

Stryker, Jeff. "Broken Promises in the AIDS War." *San Francisco Examiner,* 4 August 1994.

———. "Onan the Barbarian." *San Francisco Examiner,* 1 January 1995.

———. "Prevention of HIV Infection: Looking Back, Looking Ahead." *Journal of the American Medical Association* 273.14 (12 April 1995): 1143–8.

"Study Supports Explicit AIDS Education." *San Jose (Calif.) Mercury-News*, 17 November 1987.

Sudhoff, Karl. *The Earliest Printed Literature on Syphilis; Being Ten Tractates from the Years 1495–1498.* Florence: R. Lier, 1925.

Swadlin, Thomas. *Sermons, Meditations, and Prayers; Upon the Plague.* London: Benson, 1637.

Szasz, Thomas. *The Manufacture of Madness.* New York: Harper and Row, 1970.

"Ignore Those Subway Ads." *Tablet* (Diocese of Brooklyn, New York), 5 February 1994.

Tarczylo, Théodore. *Sexe et liberté au siècle des lumières.* Paris: Presses de la Renaissance, 1983.

Tentler, Thomas N. *Sin and Confession on the Eve of the Reformation.* Princeton: Princeton University Press, 1977.

Thomas, Keith Vivian. *Religion and the Decline of Magic: Studies in Popular Beliefs in Sixteenth- and Seventeenth-Century England.* London: Weidenfeld and Nicolson, 1971.

Tissot, Samuel-Auguste-André-David. *Avis au peuple sur la santé.* 2nd ed. Paris: Didot le Jeune, 1763.

———. *Dissertatio de febribus biliosis; seu historia epidemiae biliosae lausannensis, an. MDCCLV. Accedit tentamen de morbis ex manustupratione.* Lausanne: M.-M. Bousquet, 1758.

———. *Onanism: A Treatise upon the Disorders Produced by Masturbation: Or, the Dangerous Effects of Secret and Excessive Venery.* Translated by M. D. A. Hume. London: J. Pridden, 1766.

Torrella, Gaspare. *Tractatus cum consiliis contra pudendagram seu morbum gallicum.* In *The Earliest Printed Literature on Syphilis,* ed. Karl Sudhoff. Florence: R. Lier, 1925.

Trail, Richard R., ed. *Lives of the Fellows of the Royal College of Physicians of London, Continued to 1965.* London: Royal College of Physicians, 1968.

Trotula of Salerno (Trocta Salernitana). *De mulierum passionibus.* Edited by Clodomiro Mancini. Scientia veterum, collana di studi della cattedra di storia della medicina dell'Università di Genova 31. Genova: Università di Genova, 1962.

Trumbach, Randolph. "Sex, Gender, and Sexual Identity in Modern Culture: Male Sodomy and Female Prostitution in Enlightenment London." In *Forbidden History,* ed. John Fout, 89–106. Chicago: University of Chicago Press, 1993.

U.S. Congress. *AIDS Issues (Part I) Hearings before the Subcommittee on Health and the Environment of the Committee on Energy and Commerce,* House of Representatives. 101st Cong., 1st sess. Washington D.C.: Government Printing Office, 1984.

U.S. Department of Health and Human Services, Centers for Disease Control. "Interim Revision of Requirements for Content of AIDS-Related Written Materials." *Federal Register* 57.115 (15 June 1992): 26742–4.

U.S. Department of Labor Children's Bureau. *Infant Care.* Bureau Publication no. 8. Washington: Government Printing Office/U.S. Department of Labor, 1929.

———. *Your Child from One to Six.* Bureau Publication no. 30, rev. ed. Washington, D.C.: Government Printing Office, 1945.

United States Catholic Conference Administrative Board. "The Many Faces of AIDS: A Gospel Response." *Origins* 17.28 (December 1987): 481–9.

United States Department of Health and Human Services, PHS, CDC, *HIV/AIDS Surveillance Report* 9.2 (1999): 7–9, <http://www.cdc.gov/nchstp/hiv_aids/stats/hasr1002.pdf>.

"Vatican AIDS Meeting Hears O'Connor Assail Condom Use." *New York Times,* 14 November 1989.

V[incent], T[homas]. *God's Terrible Voice in the City of London, Wherein You Have the Narration of the Two Late Dreadful Judgements of Plague and Fire, Inflicted by the Lord upon That City, the Former in the Year 1665, the Latter in the Year 1666.* Cambridge: Samuel Green, 1667.

Van der Linden, Frank. "Disgusting Comic Book about AIDS." *Lebanon (Pa.) Daily News,* 25 October 1987.

Veith, Ilza. *Hysteria: The History of a Disease.* Chicago: University of Chicago Press, 1965.

Vincent of Beauvais (Vincent de Beauvais, Vincentius Bellovacensis). *Speculum quadruplex sive speculum maius.* Graz: Akademische Druck- u. Verlagsanstalt, 1965.

W. [Woodward, Samuel B.]. "Remarks on Masturbation"; "Insanity Produced by Masturbation";

"Effects of Masturbation with Cases." *Boston Medical and Surgical Journal* 12 (1835): 94–7; 109–12; 138–41.

Wack, Mary Frances. *Lovesickness in the Middle Ages: The* Viaticum *and Its Commentaries.* Philadelphia: University of Pennsylvania Press, 1990.

———. "The Measure of Pleasure: Peter of Spain on Men, Women, and Lovesickness." *Viator* 17 (1986): 173–96.

Webster, Charles. *The Great Instauration: Science, Medicine, and Reform, 1626–1660.* New York: Holmes and Meier, 1975.

Weiss, Rick. "President to Introduce National AIDS 'Strategy.'" *Valley News (White River Junction, Vt.; Lebanon, N.H.),* 17 December 1996.

Wendel, François. *Calvin: The Origins and Development of His Religious Thought.* Translated by Philip Mairet. New York: Harper and Row, 1963.

Wesley, John. *Primitive Physick: Or, an Easy and Natural Method of Curing Most Diseases.* 13th ed. Bristol: William Pyne, 1768 [1747].

West, Charles, M.D. "Clitoridectomy: Letter to the Editor." *Lancet,* no. 2 (17 November 1866): 560–1.

West, Mary. *Child Care, Part 1: The Preschool Age.* Care of Children Series no. 3; Bureau Publication no. 30. Washington: Government Printing Office/U.S. Department of Labor Children's Bureau, 1918.

———. *Infant Care.* Care of Children Series no. 2; Bureau Publication no. 8. Washington: Government Printing Office/U.S. Department of Labor Children's Bureau, 1914.

Who's Important in Medicine. New York: Institute for Research in Biography, 1945.

Wickersheimer, Charles. "Sur la syphilis au XVe et XVIe siècles." *Humanisme et Renaissance* 4 (1936): 157–207.

Widman (Meichinger), Johannes. *Tractatus clarissimi medicinarum Doctoris Johannis Widman dicti Meichinger, de pustulis et morbo qui vulgato nomine mal de Franzos appellatur.* In *The Earliest Printed Literature on Syphilis,* ed. Karl Sudhoff, 236–49. Florence: R. Lier, 1925.

William of Auvergne (Guillaume d'Auvergne, Guilielmus Alvernus). *De anima.* In *Opera omnia.* 2 vols. Paris: L. Billaine, 1674.

———. *De sacramento matrimonii.* In *Opera omnia,* 1: 512–27. 2 vols. Paris: L. Billaine, 1674.

William of Auxerre (Guillaume d'Auxerre, Guilielmus Altissiodorensis). *Summa Aurea.* Paris: N. Vaultier and D. Gerlier, 1500.

William of Saliceto. "Cyrurgia." In *Summa conservationis et curationis Gulielmi Placentini.* Venice: Bonetus Locatellus for Octavianus Scotus, 1502.

Wilson, Frank Percy. *The Plague in Shakespeare's London.* Oxford: Clarendon Press, 1927.

Wood, George B., M.D. *The Dispensatory of the United States of America.* 5th ed. Philadelphia: Grigg and Elliott, 1843.

———. *The Dispensatory of the United States of America.* 16th ed. Philadelphia: J. B. Lippincott Co., 1888.

Wood-Allen, Mary, M.D. *Almost a Man.* 2nd ed. Ann Arbor, Mich.: Wood-Allen Publishing Co., 1899 [1895].

———. *What a Young Girl Should Know.* Philadelphia: Vir Publishing, 1897.

Woodard, Catherine. "Cuomo Defends Archdiocese on AIDS Care." *New York Newsday,* 10 January 1990.

Woodward, Kenneth L. "Libels in the Cathedral." *Newsweek,* 1 April 1991, 59.

Zambaco, Démétrius Alexandre. "Masturbation and Psychological Problems in Two Little Girls, from *L'encéphale* 2 (1882): 88–95, 260–74." Translated by Catherine Duncan. In *A Dark Science: Women, Sexuality, and Psychiatry in the Nineteenth Century,* ed. Jeffrey Moussaieff Masson. New York: Farrar, Straus and Giroux, 1886 [1982].

———. "Onanisme avec troubles nerveux chez deux petites filles." *L'encéphale* 2 (1882): 88–95, 260–74.

Zumthor, Paul. *Histoire littéraire de la France médiévale.* Paris: Presses Universitaires de France, 1954.

INDEX